Contents

Stephanie Malherbe

ECG pocket

D1002745

www.media4u.com

Author: Prof. Ralph Haberl, Kreisklinik München-Pasing, München 81241, Germany
Editors: Ingo Haessler
Cover Illustration: Lucie Mykena, Franka Krueger
Printer: Laub GmbH & Co., Elztal-Dallau, 74834, Germany, www.laub.de
Publisher: Börm Bruckmeier Publishing LLC, www.media4u.com

IMPORTANT NOTICE - PLEASE READ!
This book is based on information from sources believed to be reliable, and every effort has been made to make the book as complete and accurate as possible and to describe generally accepted practices based on information available as of the printing date, but its accuracy and completeness cannot be guaranteed. Despite the best efforts of author and publisher, the book may contain errors, and the reader should use the book only as a general guide and not as the ultimate source of information about the subject matter.
This book is not intended to reprint all of the information available to the author or publisher on the subject, but rather to simplify, complement and supplement other available sources. The reader is encouraged to read all available material and to consult the package insert and other references to learn as much as possible about the subject.
This book is sold without warranties of any kind, expressed or implied, and the publisher and author disclaim any liability, loss or damage caused by the content of this book.
IF YOU DO NOT WISH TO BE BOUND BY THE FOREGOING CAUTIONS AND CONDITIONS , YOU MAY RETURN THIS BOOK TO THE PUBLISHER FOR A FULL REFUND.

Printed in Germany
ISBN 1-59103-202-4

Preface to the First Edition

It is tempting to buy a book that covers every single aspect of a given subject. But sometimes, after having read such a book, one does not really know much more, because of the sheer quantity of the information presented.

ECG pocket is not intended to substitute for a textbook. It was designed for medical students, residents and physicians in all specialties who need ready recognition of common ECG findings, but also want to be aware of less common ones. Concrete examples and graphics will assist them in this. This booklet does not provide expert knowledge, but rather emphasizes the importance of ECG diagnostics in primary care medicine. Those who have command of this material will be well prepared for everyday medical practice.

I will be pleased if this book can facilitate your work with patients.

Very special thanks to my assistant of many years, Regine Pulter, for her helpful contributions.

R. Haberl   Munich, December 2001

Most ECGs in this booklet are
recorded at a speed of 25 mm/sec.
Those recorded at a speed of
50 mm/sec are marked with a *.

Additional titles in this series:
Differential Diagnosis pocket
Drug pocket 2002
Medical Spanish pocket

Börm Bruckmeier Publishing LLC on the Internet:
www.media4u.com

Contents

Contents

9. Carditis,
   Cardiomyopathy

10. Electrolyte
   Disturbances, Drugs

11. Interferences and
   Artifacts

1. Basics

1.1 Conduction System

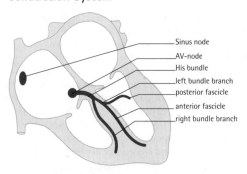

Sinus node
AV-node
His bundle
left bundle branch
posterior fascicle
anterior fascicle
right bundle branch

Fig. 1 Conduction system of the heart.

The **SA node** is the primary pacemaker of the heart. It generates a regular, electrical impulse with a frequency of 60-80 beats/min. The depolarization is then spread by way of atrial conduction pathways to the **AV node**. On passing the AV node, conduction is delayed. If the sinus node fails to function properly, the AV node can generate the impulse with a frequency of 40-60 beats/min. The depolarization then passes from the AV node through the **bundle of His** and on to the **bundle branches**. The left bundle branch divides into a left posterior and a left anterior fascicle.

1.2   ECG Waves and Intervals

The depolarization of the SA node cannot be seen in the ECG. Atrial depolarization is represented by **P waves**. The first phase of the P wave corresponds to depolarization of the right atrium; depolarization of the left atrium follows.

Atrial repolarization cannot be seen because it coincides with the **QRS complex**. At the end of the P wave the atria are completely depolarized and the impulse spreads by way of the AV node to the bundle of His. The **Q wave** represents the depolarization of the septum and the impulse quickly continues by way of the Purkinje fibers to the ventricles. At the end of the QRS complex the ventricles are completely depolarized. Due to the electromechanical delay, ventricular contraction starts at the end of the QRS complex. The normal **ST segment** is isoelectric and begins at the end of the S wave.

Ventricular repolarization produces the **T wave**. The significance of the **U wave** is unknown.

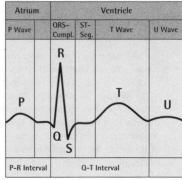

Atrium		Ventricle			
P Wave	QRS–Compl.	ST–Seg.	T Wave	U Wave	
P-R Interval		Q-T Interval			

Fig. 2
ECG waves and intervals.

1.3   The ECG Leads

The standard ECG consists of the following leads

1. Einthoven's extremity (limb) leads (I, II, III)

These are bipolar leads. The amplitude is positive if the depolarization moves towards the positive electrode marked with +.

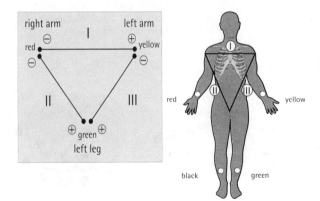

Fig. 3 Einthoven's triangle of the limb leads.
Fig. 4 Placement of the limb leads.

2. Wilson's chest (precordial) leads (V_1 – V_6)

These leads are unipolar. They measure the voltage of any one electrode relative to a constructed zero potential.
The electrodes are placed as follows:

V_1	fourth intercostal space to the right of the sternum
V_2	fourth intercostal space to the left of the sternum
V_3	midway between V_2 and V_4
V_4	fifth intercostal space in the left midclavicular line
V_5	fifth intercostal space in the left anterior axillary line
V_6	fifth intercostal space in the left midaxillary line

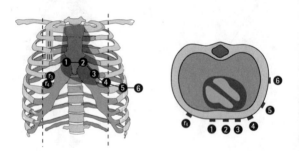

Fig. 5 Placement of the unipolar chest leads (left) and reflection of the heart seen in a cross section (right).

Caution

Placing the electrodes improperly, for example in the second intercostal space, may lead to an R reduction in the anterior leads and may, therefore, be misinterpreted as an old anterior myocardial infarction.

If a right ventricular infarction is suspected, Vr4 on the right side of the chest is useful.

3. Goldberger's augmented leads (aVR, aVL, aVF)

The augmented leads are obtained by recording voltages from the limbs. Their amplitudes are higher. The "a" stands for "augmented".

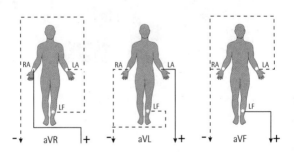

Fig. 6 Augmented leads.

Localization of a myocardial infarction

Particularly in the diagnosis of a myocardial infarction, the localization of the pathological event seen in the reflecting leads is important. Guidelines are summarized in the following figure.

Infarct Localization										
	I	II	III	aVL	aVF	rV4	V2	V3	V4	V5	V6
apical	+			+			+	+	+		
anteroseptal							+	+			
anterolateral	+			+						+	+
posterolateral			+		+					+	+
inferior		+	+		+						
right ventricular			+		+	+	(+)				

Fig. 7 Infarct localization.

1.4 Methods

The paper usually moves at a **speed** of 50 mm/sec. with an amplification of 1 mV/cm. Thus, 1 cm on the paper corresponds to 200 ms = 0.2 s.
Most ECGs in this booklet are recorded at a speed of 25 mm/sec; those recorded at a speed of 50 mm/sec are marked with a *.

The **heart rate** is determined using the following formula:

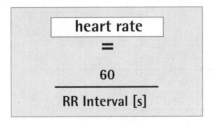

$$\text{heart rate} = \frac{60}{\text{RR Interval [s]}}$$

Fig. 8 Calculation of heart rate.

2. The Normal ECG

2.1 Characteristics of the Normal ECG

Recognizing a pathological ECG is half the battle.
The **normal intervals** are shown in **Fig. 9**.

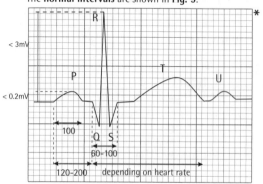

Fig. 9 Normal intervals of the ECG: P wave < 100ms,
PR interval < 200ms, QRS complex < 100ms.

All ECG intervals should be measured in the lead showing the
biggest aberration.
The P wave and the QRS complex should not take longer than
100 ms, the PR interval not longer than 200 ms.
The QT interval depends on the heart rate. A prolonged QT interval
caused by a congenital long QT syndrome or secondary to drugs (p.
214), can cause severe cardiac arrhythmias.

Fig. 10 shows standard values for the QT interval depending on the heart rate including lower and upper limits. A prolongation of the PR interval is called a "first degree heart block," a prolonged QRS complex a "bundle branch block."

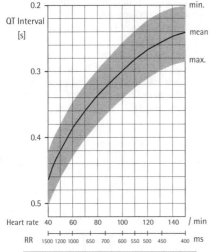

Bazett Formula: $QT_c = \dfrac{QT\ [s]}{\sqrt{RR\ [s]}}$

(n = 0.40 – 0.44)

Fig. 10 Normogram of QT interval. Mean value and tolerance range. Waves in seconds. RR: interval between two Rs.

2.2   Axis Determination

The cardiac axis reflects the electrical axis of the average direction of the ventricular activation in the frontal plane as the depolarization wave spreads through the ventricles. The cardiac axis is derived from the QRS complex in leads I, II and III. A useful system for the determination of the cardiac axis is demonstrated in **Fig. 12**.

The normal cardiac axis of an adolescent shows an angle of +30° to +90°, that of an adult of -30° to +60°. It is not the maximum amplitude of a single lead that is important when calculating the cardiac axis, but the mean QRS vector, including all positive and negative deflections (**Fig. 11**).

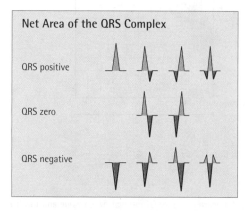

Fig. 11 Axis: determination of the QRS net area.

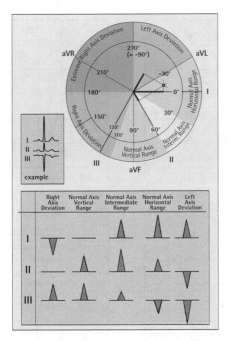

Fig. 12 Cardiac axis and Lewis circle. **For example** the positive QRS deflection is transferred to leads I, II and III. If it is negative, the arrow points away from that lead. Lines through the head of the arrows and perpendicular to the leads cross in one point of the circle demonstrating the cardiac axis.

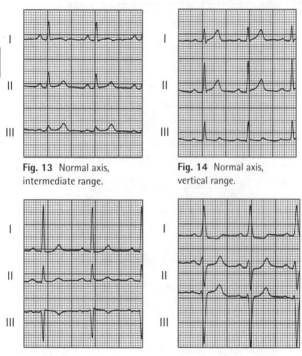

Fig. 13 Normal axis, intermediate range.

Fig. 14 Normal axis, vertical range.

Fig. 15 Normal axis, horizontal range.

Fig. 16 Left axis deviation.

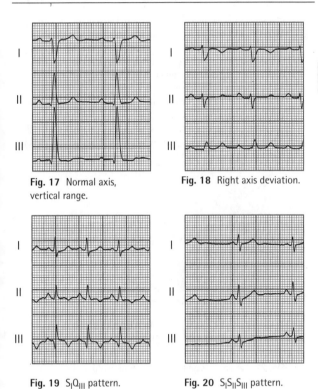

Fig. 17 Normal axis, vertical range.

Fig. 18 Right axis deviation.

Fig. 19 S$_I$Q$_{III}$ pattern.

Fig. 20 S$_I$S$_{II}$S$_{III}$ pattern.

Changes in the cardiac axis can be caused by muscular hypertrophy (normal axis vertical range due to hypertension, normal axis horizontal range due to right ventricular hypertrophy), by changes in the anatomic position of the heart and by disorders of conduction (for example bundle branch block, fascicular block, p. 43). A left anterior fascicular block (p. 48) leads to a left axis deviation, a left posterior fascicular block to right axis deviation. Typical cardiac axes show aberrations in the frontal plane. Shifting and rotation of the heart in the sagittal and horizontal planes (**Fig. 20**) lead to $S_I Q_{III}$ or $S_I S_{II} S_{III}$ patterns. Both of these axis deviations can be a sign of strain on the right ventricle.

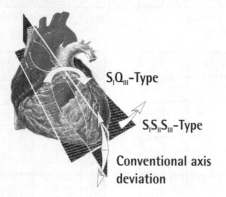

$S_I Q_{III}$-Type

$S_I S_{II} S_{III}$-Type

Conventional axis deviation

Fig. 21 Cardiac axis and special types of axis deviation.

2.3   Evaluation of the ECG

A systematic method for reading and interpreting an ECG should be developed and the following features should be analyzed. Although some of them may require a more detailed knowledge of ECG, they are mentioned here in order to provide guidelines for complete ECG interpretation. The single steps of ECG analysis are as follows:

1. Rhythm
The regularity of the rhythm is determined by assessing the **RR intervals**. **Tachycardia** is an increased heart rate > 90 beats/min. In **bradycardia** the heart rate is less than 50 beats/min. Sinus rhythm is defined by regular positive **P waves** in I - III.

2. Atrioventricular conduction
In a normal AV conduction the time from the start of the P wave to the start of the QRS complex is < 200 ms. Therefore the **PR interval** is < 0.2 s. Otherwise it demonstrates an AV block.

3. Axis
The cardiac axis is assessed as mentioned above, using the pattern shown in **Fig. 12**.

4. QRS complex
A normal QRS complex duration is 100 ms. A QRS complex that takes > 100 ms is a sign of a bundle branch block. In the chest leads the R amplitude increases constantly from V_1 to V_6 (the so-called R progression). A decrease in the R amplitude is possible in V_5 and V_6 due to a longer distance between those leads and the chest wall. While interpreting the QRS complex, special attention must be paid to significant Q waves and signs of cardiac hypertrophy.

5. ST segment

In a normal ECG the ST segment is isoelectric. An insignificant ST elevation may occur only in V_2 and V_3 (up to 0.2 mV). Changes in the ST segment may be found in myocardial ischemia.

6. T wave

The T waves in leads I - III and V_1 - V_6 are always positive. A negative T wave in a chest lead is always pathologic with the following exception: T waves in V_1 and III may be slightly negative.

7. QT interval

The next step is to assess the QT interval. By using the corrected QT interval (QTc) a predisposition to cardiac arrhythmias can be recognized.

8. Presumption diagnosis

At the end of an ECG analysis a presumption diagnosis should be made keeping the clinical picture of the patient in mind.

The following diagram shows an **ECG evaluation sheet**.
This evaluation sheet is available as a plastic card, **ECG Evaluation pocketcard**. It can also be found in the appendix of this book or on the Internet under **www.media4u.com**. It can be copied or downloaded and used for your own ECG interpretations.

ECG Evaluation Sheet

Patient
- Initials ___ Date of birth |_day_|_month_| 1 , 9 |___| Sex F M
- Main diagnosis: ___
- Antiarrhythmics: ___ Digitalis ○

RR Intervals Regular Y N

Heart Rate ___ / min Tachycardia (> 90/min) ○ Bradycardia (< 50/min) ○

P Wave
- Positive in I, II, III (sinus rhythm) Y N
- Regular, followed by QRS Y N — absolute arrhythmia (atrial fibrillation) ○
  "sawtooth" (atrial flutter) ○

PR Interval 0.12 – 0.20 s Y N — shortened, < 0.12 s ○ prolonged, > 0.2 s (AV block) ○

Axis Deviation
- $S_I Q_{III}$ pattern ○ $(S_I S_{II} S_{III}$ pattern) ○ Extreme axis deviation ○
  Left axis deviation ○ Right axis deviation ○
- Normal ○

QRS Complex QRS duration normal < 0.1 s Y N—
- Incomplete bundle branch block (0.10 – 0.12 s) ○
- Complete bundle branch block (> 0.12 s) ○
- Terminal deflection delayed in V_1 (> 0.03 s)← RBBB ○
- Terminal deflection delayed in V_6 (> 0.05 s)← LBBB ○

R Progression Normal in $V_1 – V_6$ Y N — insufficient R Progression in V_1 ○ V_2 ○ V_3 ○ V_4 ○ V_5 ○ V_6 ○

Q Wave Significantly pathological in N Y V_1 ○ V_2 ○ V_3 ○ V_4 ○ V_5 ○ V_6 ○ II ○ III ○ aVF ○

Signs of Hypertrophy N Y $S_{V2} + R_{V5}$ > 3.5 mV (Sokolov le.)○ $R_{V2} + S_{V5}$ > 1.05 mV (Sokolov ri.) ○

ST Segment Isoelectric Y N — ST elevation in V_1 ○ V_2 ○ V_3 ○ V_4 ○ V_5 ○ V_6 ○ I ○ II III ○ aVR aVL aVF ○
- ST depression in V_1 ○ V_2 ○ V_3 ○ V_4 ○ V_5 ○ V_6 ○ I ○ II III ○ aVR aVL aVF ○
- ascend. ○ horizont. ○ descend. ○

T Wave Positive in I - III, V_1–V_4 Y N — negative T wave symmetr. ○ preterminal ○ terminal ○

QT Interval QT_C normal (0.40-0.44) Y N QT interval: |_._| Corrected QT interval (QT_C) |_._| Bazett: $\frac{QT (s)}{\sqrt{RR (s)}}$

Evaluation (ECG Diagnosis) Normal ○ Borderline ○ Pathological ○

© 1997–2002
Börm Bruckmeier Publishing LLC
www.media4u.com

Signature ___ Date |_month_|_day_| 2 , 0 |___|

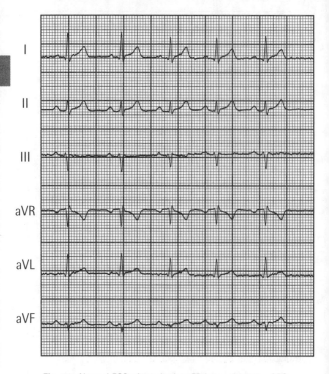

Fig. 22 Normal ECG: sinus rhythm, PR interval < 0.2 s, QRS complex < 0.1 s, normal axis, horizontal range.

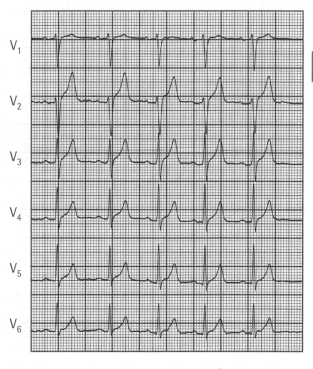

Normal R progression, isoelectric ST segment (up to 0.2 mV in V_2 is normal), T wave is positive in all chest leads.

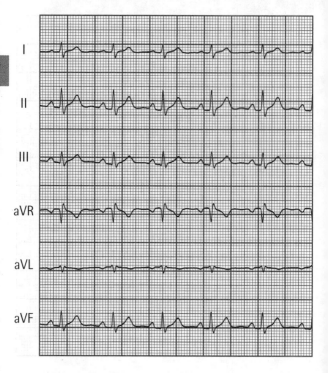

Fig. 23 Normal ECG. Normal cardiac axis, intermediate range (+60° to +90°)

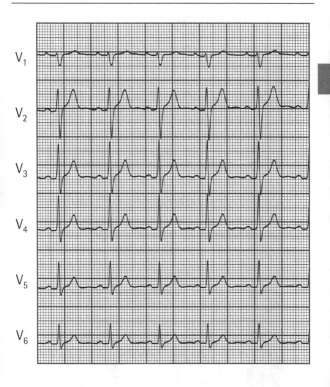

2.4 Normal Pediatric ECG Values

Age	Heart Rate (min⁻¹)	QRS Axis (Axis Deviation)	PR Interval (s)	QRS Complex (s)	R in V₁ (mm)	S in V₁ (mm)	R in V₆ (mm)	S in V₆ (mm)
1 wk	90–160	60°–180°	0.08–0.15	0.03–0.08	5–26	0–23	0–12	0–10
2–3 wk	100–180	45°–160°	0.08–0.15	0.03–0.08	3–21	0–16	2–16	0–10
4–8 wk	120–180	30°–135°	0.08–0.15	0.03–0.08	3–18	0–15	5–21	0–10
3–5 mo	105–185	0°–135°	0.08–0.15	0.03–0.08	3–20	0–15	6–22	0–10
6–12 mo	110–170	0°–135°	0.07–0.16	0.03–0.08	2–20	0.5–20	6–23	0–7
2 yr	90–165	0°–110°	0.08–0.16	0.03–0.08	2–18	0.5–21	6–23	0–7
3–4 yr	70–140	0°–110°	0.09–0.17	0.04–0.08	1–18	0.5–21	4–24	0–5
5–7 yr	65–140	0°–110°	0.09–0.17	0.04–0.08	0.5–14	0.5–24	4–26	0–4
8–11 yr	60–130	–15°–110°	0.09–0.17	0.04–0.09	0.5–14	0.5–25	4–25	0–4
12–15 yr	65–130	–15°–110°	0.09–0.18	0.04–0.09	0–14	0.5–21	4–25	0–4
> 16 yr	50–120	–15°–110°	0.12–0.20	0.05–0.10	0–14	0.5–23	4–21	0–4

3.   Hypertrophy of the Heart

3.1   Right Atrial Enlargement

P-pulmonale

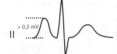

Elevated, peaked P wave > 0.2 mV, particularly in II, III and aVF as a sign of right atrial hypertrophy. The PR interval is not considerably prolonged. Frequently associated with signs of right ventricular hypertrophy or vertical range cardiac axis ($S_I Q_{III}$ type).

Etiology
Often a sign of volume or pressure overload of the right atrium, for example in tricuspid insufficiency, atrial septal defect or pulmonary hypertension.

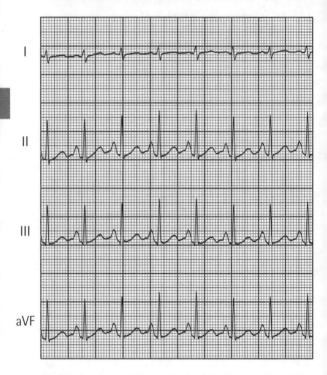

Fig. 24 P-pulmonale. The amplitude of the P wave in II and III is > 0.2 mV, the duration of the P wave is normal (< 0.1 s).

3.2   Left Atrial Enlargement

P-mitrale

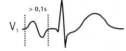

Widening of the P wave > 0.1 s, particularly in I, II and V_1 - V_3 as a sign of left atrial hypertrophy.

A **biphasic P** wave with a marked negative deflection in V_1 is frequently found and is often associated with signs of left ventricular hypertrophy.

Causes

P-mitrale is a sign of pressure or volume overload of the left atrium, for example in mitral stenosis or mitral regurgitation.

3.3 Right Ventricular Hypertrophy

Definition
Thickening of the right ventricular muscle as a response to chronic volume or pressure overload.

ECG
A very common index for ventricular hypertrophy is the Sokolow index. In right ventricular hypertrophy the Sokolow index is positive: R in V_2 + S in V_5 > 1.05 mV.
Further criteria are listed in **Fig. 25**.
RVH is frequently associated with repolarization disorders in V_1 - V_3, vertical range cardiac axis ($S_I Q_{III}$ type) and P-pulmonale.

Causes
RVH is a sign of volume or pressure overload of the right ventricle (**Fig. 26**).

Right Ventricular Hypertrophy

- R wave in V_1	> 0.7 mV
- R wave in V_2 + S wave in V_5 (Sokolov-Lyon)	> 1.05 mV
- R/S ratio in V_1	> 1
- R/S ratio in V_5 or V_6	< 1

- S_I-Q_{III}-type, sagittal-type
- right axis deviation
- right bundle branch block
- P waves: tall and peaked

Fig. 25 ECG Criteria of right ventricular hypertrophy.

Right Ventricular Hypertrophy

- Primary pulmonary disease
- Pulmonary stenosis
- Tetralogy of Fallot
- Mitral valve disease with pulmonary hypertension
- Sleep apnea
- Eisenmenger's syndrome
- Pulmonary emboli

Fig. 26 Possible causes of right ventricular hypertrophy.

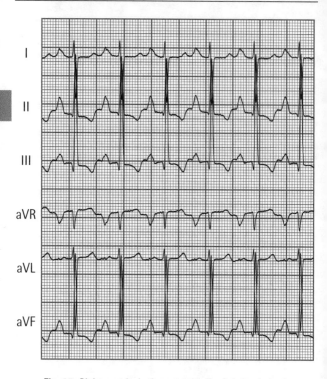

Fig. 27 Right ventricular hypertrophy. The Sokolow index is pathological: R in V_2 + S in V_5 are > 1.05 mV.

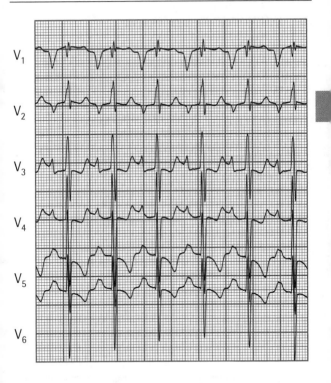

3.4 Left Ventricular Hypertrophy

Definition

Thickening of the left ventricular muscle as a response to chronic pressure or volume overload (hypertension, aortic stenosis).

ECG

A very common index for ventricular hypertrophy is the Sokolow index. With left ventricular hypertrophy the Sokolow index is positive: S in V_2 + the R in V_5 > 3.5 mV.

Further criteria in **Fig. 30**. These criteria are not valid in combination with a left branch bundle block.

Causes

See **Fig. 31**.

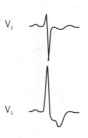

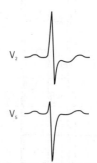

Fig. 28 Left ventricular hypertrophy.

Fig. 29 Right ventricular hypertrophy.

Left Ventricular Hypertrophy

- R wave in I	> 1.6 mV
- R wave in I + S wave in III	> 2.5 mV
(Gubner u. Ungerleider)	
- R wave in V_4, V_5 or V_6	> 2.6 mV
- R wave in V_5 oder V_6 + S wave in V_1 or V_2	> 3.5 mV
(Sokolov-Lyon)	

- QRS duration > 80 ms
- P waves: broadened > 0.1 s
- left axis deviation
- impaired P wave progression V_1 - V_3

Fig. 30 ECG Criteria of Left ventricular hypertrophy.

Left Ventricular Hypertrophy

- Systemic hypertension
- Aortic stenosis
- Hypertrophic cardiomyopathy

Fig. 31 Possible causes of Left ventricular hypertrophy.

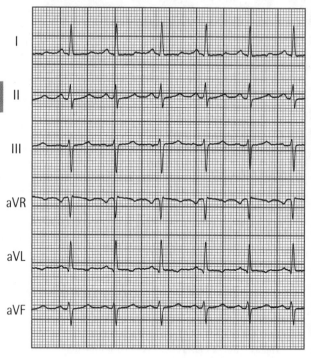

Fig. 32 Left ventricular overload: S in V_2 + R in V_5 > 3.5 mV. Often a reduced R progression is found, in rare cases a left axis deviation.

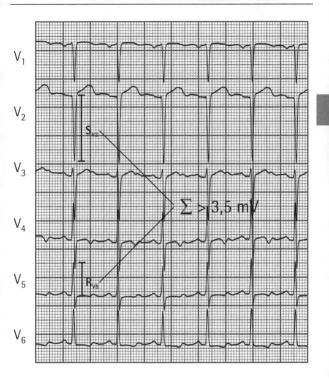

4. Bundle Branch Block

4.1 General Description

Definition
Conduction disturbances in the His bundle or in one of the bundle branches.

Anatomy

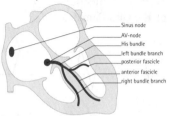

Fig. 33   Conduction system of the heart.

Forms
Complete or incomplete bundle branch block.
RBBB, LBBB, left anterior or left posterior fascicular block,
functional bundle branch block,
bifascicular block, trifascicular block.

ECG
Widening of the QRS complex > 0.12 s in a complete bundle branch block. A QRS complex of > 0.10 and < 0.12 s is a sign of an incomplete bundle branch block.

To determine if a right or left bundle branch block is present, the start of the **negative terminal deflection** is used. It is defined as the last negative deflection in the QRS complex. Terminal negativity is delayed in V_1 in a right bundle branch block, in V_6 in a left bundle branch block and in both in an arborization block (rare, found only in severe heart disease).

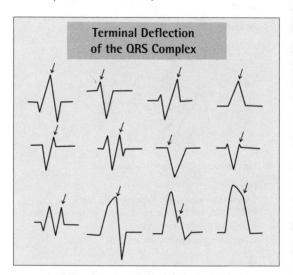

Fig. 34 Determination of the terminal deflection of the QRS complex, defined as the last negative deflection in the QRS complex.

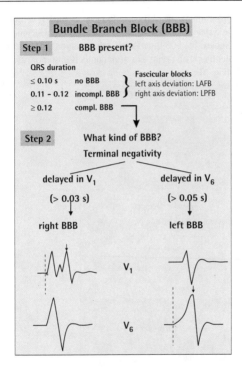

Bundle Branch Block (BBB)

Step 1   BBB present?

QRS duration
≤ 0.10 s   no BBB   Fascicular blocks
0.11 – 0.12   incompl. BBB   left axis deviation: LAFB
≥ 0.12   compl. BBB   right axis deviation: LPFB

Step 2   What kind of BBB?
                  Terminal negativity

delayed in V₁   delayed in V₆

(> 0.03 s)   (> 0.05 s)

right BBB   left BBB

V₁

V₆

Fig. 35 Evaluation of bundle branch blocks. A complete BBB is present, when QRS > 0.12 s. The type of BBB is diagnosed by determining the lead with a delay of the terminal deflection.

An interruption of one of the two fascicles of the left ventricular Purkinje system leads to a fascicular block without widening of the QRS complex. The ECG shows a left axis deviation (left anterior fascicular block) or a right axis deviation (left posterior fascicular block) (**Fig. 36**).

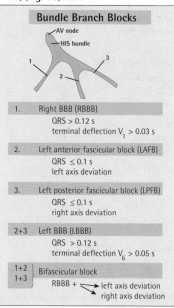

Fig. 36 Forms of bundle branch block (BBB).

Causes

Causes of bundle branch blocks are shown in the following diagram
(**Fig. 37**).

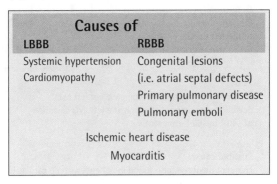

Fig. 37 Possible causes of bundle branch blocks.

4.2   Left Anterior Fascicular Block

Definition
Block of the anterior fascicle
of the left bundle branch
(left anterior fascicular block).

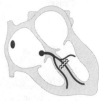

Left anterior fascicular block

ECG
No broadening of the QRS complex, but left axis
deviation. The diagnosis is likely if a left axis deviation
of -40 ° to -60 ° is present.

Possible causes
Frequent diagnosis, also found in patients with no cardiac history.

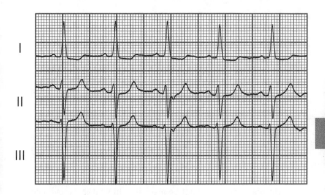

Fig. 38 Left anterior fascicular block. Left axis deviation.
The QRS complex is normal.

4.3 Left Posterior Fascicular Block

Definition
Block of the posterior fascicle
of the left bundle branch
(left posterior fascicular block).

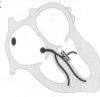

Left posterior fascicular block

ECG
No widening of the QRS complex, but right axis deviation.

Caution
The diagnosis should not be made if right ventricular overload,
pulmonary emphysema or a posterolateral infarction is present.

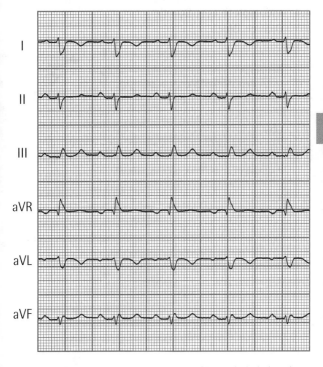

Fig. 39 Left posterior fascicular block. Right axis deviation, the QRS complex is normal.

4.4 Incomplete Left Bundle Branch Block

Definition
Incomplete block of the left bundle branch.

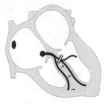

Incomplete left bundle branch block

ECG
Widening of the QRS complex > 0.10 s, but < 0.12 s.
The R amplitude is reduced over the anterior wall, so the exact diagnosis of an ischemic event is difficult.

4.5 Complete Left Bundle Branch Block

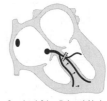

Complete left bundle branch block

Definition
Complete conduction block in the main division of the LBB.

ECG
Widening of the QRS complex > 0.12 s and a delay of terminal negativity in V_6 of > 0.05 s. One of the main characteristics is the complete **loss of the R wave** on the anterior wall. This must not be interpreted as an old anterior myocardial infarction! Further signs are left precordial repolarization disturbances and ST segment elevations.

Caution
In the presence of an LBBB there is no conclusive way to diagnose an acute myocardial infarction or instable angina except to compare the ECG with an old one. ST changes seen during an exercise stress test have no diagnostic value with a preexisting LBBB.

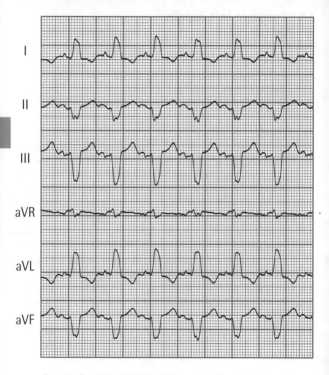

Fig. 40 Complete LBBB. The QRS complex is > 0.12 s,
the terminal deflection is delayed in V_6 > 0.05 s,

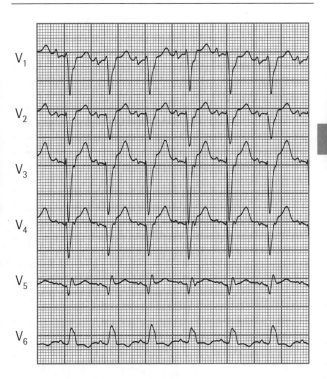

typical R loss on the anterior wall and secondary repolarization disturbances.

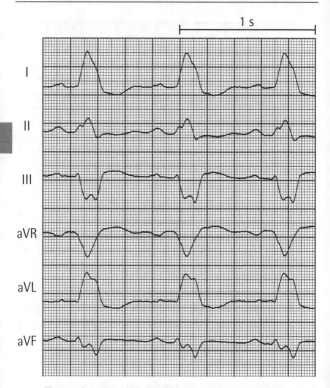

Fig. 41 Complete LBBB. The QRS complex is > 0.12 s, the terminal deflection is delayed > 0.05 s in V_6. There is an R loss over

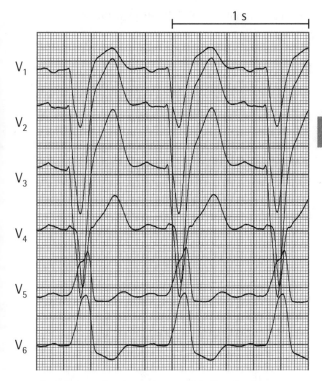

the anterior wall and secondary repolarization disorders.
Caution: written at a speed of 50 mm/s.

4.6   Functional Left Bundle Branch Block

Definition
Intermittent occurrence of an LBBB.

ECG
The ECG shows a sinus rhythm with an intermittent widening of the QRS complex of > 0.12 s, a delay of terminal negativity in V_6 and an R loss in the anterior leads.

Causes
The most common cause is the frequency-dependent intermittent LBBB, for example in an exercise tolerance test, but it is also associated with coronary heart disease.

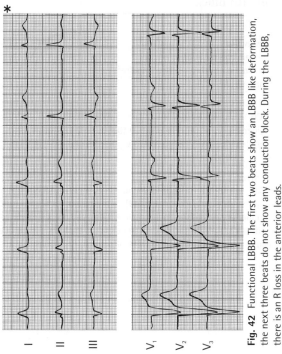

*

I

II

III

V₁

V₂

V₃

Fig. 42 Functional LBBB. The first two beats show an LBBB like deformation, the next three beats do not show any conduction block. During the LBBB, there is an R loss in the anterior leads.

4.7 Incomplete Right Bundle Branch Block

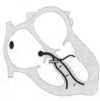

Definition
Incomplete interruption of the conduction of the electrical impulse through the RBBB.

Incomplete right bundle branch block

ECG
Widening of the QRS complex > 0.10 s, but < 0.12 s, delay in terminal negativity of > 0.03 s in V_1, often R prime (R′) in V_1.

Causes
May be a normal variation in young adults, otherwise it is a sign of right ventricular overload (**Fig. 43**). In the case of an acute **pulmonary embolism**, an incomplete RBBB may occur, associated with an S_IQ_{III}-type, tachycardia and clinical symptoms. Typical ECG signs are only seen in approx. 20% of pulmonary embolism cases.

Right Ventricular Overload

ECG Criteria

- P waves: tall and peaked
- Right axis deviation
- Right ventricular hypertrophy
- (Incomplete) right BBB
- Secondary: ST and T wave abnormalities in V_1, V_2

Causes

- Primary pulmonary disease
- Pulmonary stenosis
- Tetralogy of Fallot
- Mitral valve disease with pulmonary hypertension
- Sleep apnea
- Eisenmenger's syndrome
- Pulmonary emboli

Fig. 43 Right ventricular overload.

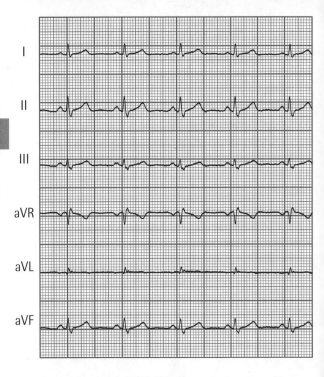

Fig. 44 Incomplete RBBB. The QRS complex is prolonged to 0.11 s and an rSr′ complex can be seen in V₁.

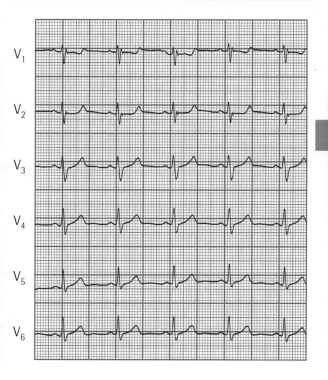

4.8 Complete Right Bundle Branch Block

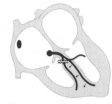

Complete right bundle branch block

Definition
Conduction through the right bundle branch is completely obstructed.

ECG
Broadening of the QRS complex > 0.12 s and delay in terminal negativity > 0.03 s. A rSr' complex is common in V_1 and repolarization disorders in V_1 - V_3 are often present.

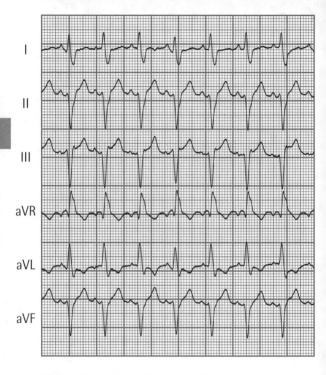

Fig. 45 Complete RBBB. The QRS complex is > 0.12 s, terminal negativity is delayed in V_1 and secondary repolarization disorders

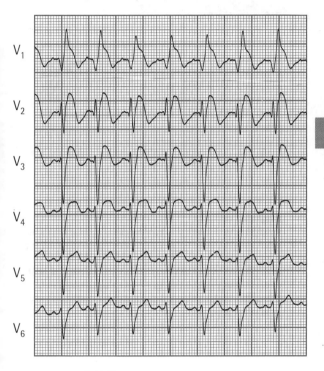

are present in V_1-V_3.

4.9   Bifascicular Block

Definition
Combination of a complete RBBB
and a LAFB (left anterior fascicular
block) or a LPFB (left posterior
fascicular block)
(**Fig. 46**).

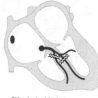

Bifascicular block

The ECG signs do not prove a bifascicular block diagnosis,
but they indicate that it is likely.

Cause
Frequently there is a severe underlying cardiac disease.

Prognosis
An RBBB with an LPFB has a poor prognosis because the residual
anterior bundle branch is very vulnerable. The combination of a
bifascicular block with a first degree AV block also has a poor
prognosis. If a trifascicular block develops, there is a danger of
cardiac arrest (asystole). Due to the severe underlying cardiac
disease, the implantation of a pacemaker does not remarkably
improve the prognosis.

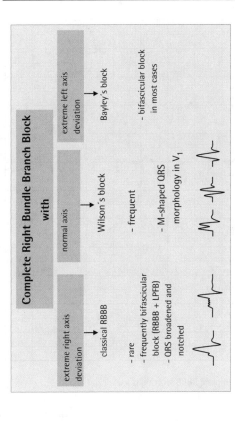

Fig. 46 Forms of an RBBB. RBBB with axis deviation is indicative of a bifascicular block.

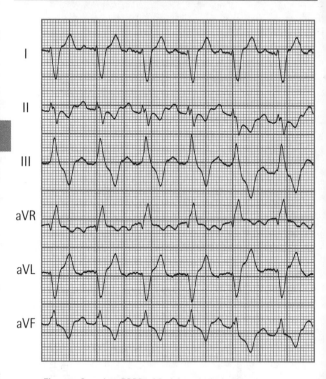

Fig. 47 Complete RBBB with right axis deviation.
A bifascicular block with a conduction defect in the

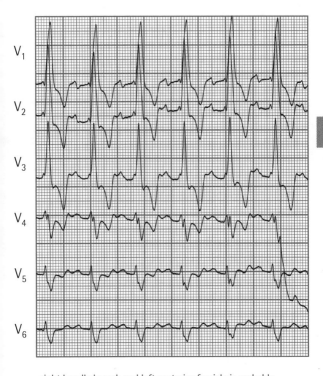

right bundle branch and left posterior fascicle is probable (classical RBBB).

5. Atrio-Ventricular Block

5.1 General Description

Definition
Conduction disturbances between
the atria and the ventricles.

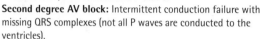

AV block

Classification of AV blocks
First degree AV block: Consistent delay
in conduction, the PR interval is > 0.20 s.
Second degree AV block: Intermittent conduction failure with
missing QRS complexes (not all P waves are conducted to the
ventricles).
Third degree AV block: Complete conduction block of all electrical
impulses between atria and ventricles. Atria and ventricles beat
independently.

Possible causes of AV-block
• Coronary artery disease
• Atrial septal defect
• Myocarditis, Endocarditis
• Sarcoidosis of the heart
• Drugs   Betablockers
Calcium antagonists (Verapamil type)
Digitalis, Adenosine
• Congenital forms

Fig. 48
Causes of AV
block.

5.2 First Degree AV Block

> 0,2s

Definition
Delay in conduction at the AV node or His bundle.

ECG
The PR interval is > 0.20 s.
Every P wave is followed by a QRS complex.

Prognosis
A first degree AV block does not cause symptoms and does not explain vertigo or fainting. However, it may lead to a higher degree of AV block. In that case a 24-hour ECG or even a His bundle electrocardiogram are indicated (**Fig. 49**). The prolongation of the AH interval has a good prognosis, prolongation of the HV interval > 80 ms may predispose to a third degree AV block.

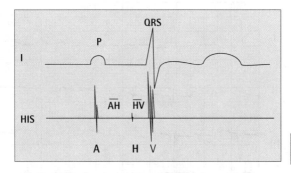

Fig. 49 His bundle electrocardiography. An electrode catheter is placed in the right ventricle and pulled back until the His signal can be recorded. The PR interval consists of the AH interval and the HV interval.

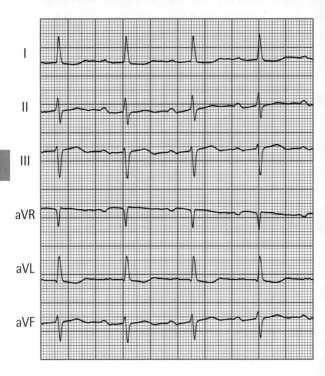

Fig. 50 First degree AV block. The PR interval is 0.34 s; every P wave is followed by a QRS complex.

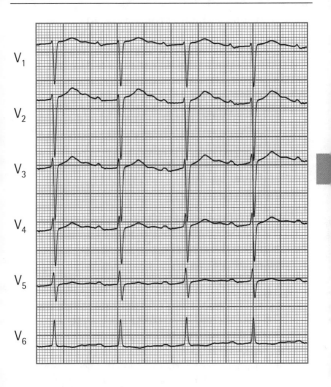

5.3   2° AV Block Mobitz I (Wenckebach)

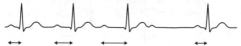

ECG

Progressive prolongation of the PR interval until a P wave is blocked and the QRS complex is dropped. The AH interval increases constantly, whereas the RR interval progressively shortens. The HV interval remains normal.

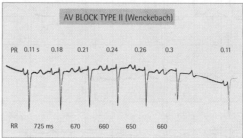

Fig. 51 2° AV Block, Mobitz type I (Wenckebach). PR interval is progressively prolonged whereas RR intervals shorten until ventricular conduction drops.

Prognosis

The prognosis is good, rarely leading to a third degree AV block. It can be seen as a normal variant in healthy patients with an increased vagus tone (while sleeping). It is not an indication for the implantation of a pacemaker.

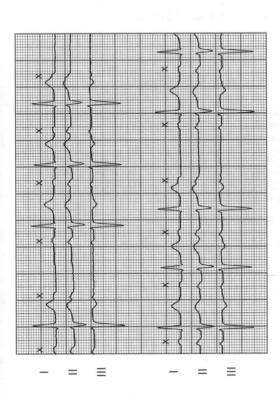

Fig. 52 Second degree AV block, type 1 (Wenckebach). The PR interval is progressively prolonged until the P wave is no longer conducted to the ventricle. P waves marked with X.

5.4   2° AV Block Mobitz Type II

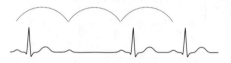

Definition

Intermittent failure of the AV conduction, the PR interval remains within normal limits.

ECG

Intermittent drop of a ventricular complex. The PR interval is constant and within normal limits. The underlying event is the prolongation of the HV interval.

Prognosis

Frequent progression to third degree AV block. In most cases this is an indication for pacemaker implantation.

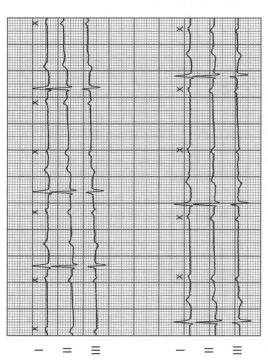

Fig. 53 Second degree AV block, Mobitz type II. The PR interval is within normal limits with an intermittent drop of conduction to the ventricles. P waves marked with X.

5.5 Third Degree AV Block

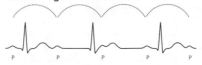

Definition
Complete block of the AV conduction.

ECG
Atria and ventricles beat independently, with no relation between P waves and QRS complexes. There is no AV conduction; the ventricular depolarization is paced by an **escape mechanism** (p. 125), which can be localized in the bundle of His (small QRS complex) or in the ventricle (BBB-like ventricular complex). Failure of the ventricular escape rhythm can lead to an asystole (Adams-Stokes attack) still showing regular P waves.

Causes
A third-degree AV block occurs as a complication of posterior myocardial infarction (occlusion of the artery supplying the AV node) and in bacterial endocarditis (abscess in the septum, see also **Fig. 48**, p. 73).

Treatment
Third degree AV block is an absolute indication for pacemaker placement except in an old AV block with a stable escape rhythm. In patients with atrial fibrillation and a fast ventricular rate, a catheter ablation of the bundle of His with a consecutive third degree AV block might be an alternative treatment. These patients need subsequent pacemaker placement.

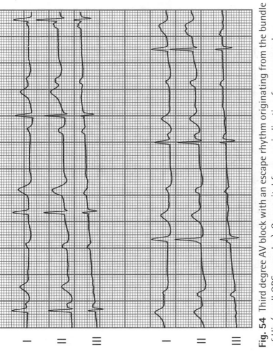

I
II
III

I
II
III

Fig. 54 Third degree AV block with an escape rhythm originating from the bundle of His (small QRS complex). Congenital form, no indication for a pacemaker.

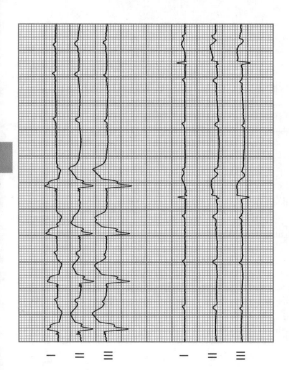

—   =   ≡   —   =   ≡

Fig. 55 Third degree AV block. After the ventricular pacemaker is switched off, only P waves are visible until two narrow ventricular QRS complexes (possibly originating from the bundle of His) occur. The ST elevation in II and III indicates an acute posterior myocardial infarction as the cause of the AV block.

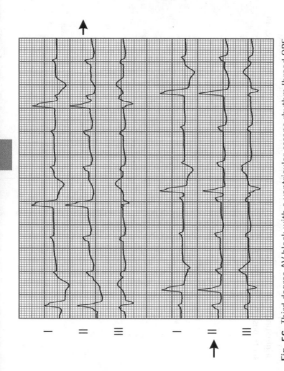

Fig. 56 Third degree AV block with a ventricular escape rhythm (broad QRS complexes).

6. Myocardial Ischemia

Basics

The coronary arteries are located in the subepicardium, so the inner part of the ventricular wall, the subendocardium, is very vulnerable to ischemia. (**Fig. 57**)

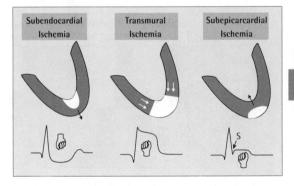

Fig. 57 Forms of myocardial ischemia. Subendocardial ischemia is caused by coronary stenosis and results in ST depression. Transmural ischemia represents acute myocardial infarction and is characterized by monophasic ST elevation. Subepicardial ischemia may be caused by pericarditis. ST elevation then frequently evolves from the S wave.

Subendocardial ischemia is a sign of hypoperfusion caused by coronary artery stenosis during times of increased demand like physical or mental stress.

The ECG in subendocardial ischemia shows ST depression. An acute myocardial infarction leads to transmural ischemia with ST elevation (**Fig. 58**).

Infarct Localization											
	I	II	III	aVL	aVF	rV4	V2	V3	V4	V5	V6
apical	+			+			+	+	+		
anteroseptal							+	+			
anterolateral	+			+						+	+
posterolateral			+		+					+	+
inferior		+	+		+						
right ventricular			+		+	+	(+)				

Fig. 58 Infarct localization, reflecting leads (12-lead ECG)

Pericarditis causes epicardial damage and leads to ST elevation originating from the S wave.

Diagnostic problems

Ischemic damage does not necessarily lead to ECG changes. It depends on the size and site of the affected area. Approx. 4% of all myocardial infarcts are silent, meaning there are no changes in the ECG. Posterior MIs often present a diagnostic challenge since they are only evident in the limb leads. Septal MIs may be difficult to diagnose because ST elevations of up to 2 mm in $V_1 - V_2$ may be normal variants. The evaluation of right sided MIs may require right sided chest leads (Vr4).

6.1 Ischemia in Coronary Artery Disease

Clinical picture

Significant coronary stenosis is defined as the occlusion of > 75% of a coronary artery which can lead to myocardial ischemia resulting in angina, especially during physical activity or in cold weather. Myocardial ischemia can also be asymptomatic or silent.

ECG

Subendocardial ischemia typically leads to horizontal or descending ST depression in the reflecting leads.
Ascending ST depressions are only pathologic if > 0.1 mV.

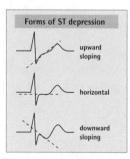
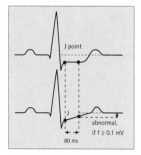

Fig. 59 Forms of ST depression: Upward sloping ST depression is a normal finding which may occur with strong physical activity. Horizontal and down sloping ST depressions are typical for myocardial ischemia.
Fig. 60 J point.

An ascending ST depression is considered abnormal, if the depression is still > 0.1 mV 80 ms after the J point (**Fig. 60**). An ascending ST depression is a normal finding during vigorous physical activity, such as an exercise stress test. This is an important aspect in the interpretation of exercise stress tests. After the exercise is stopped, the ST depressions resolve within minutes. **Prinzmetal angina**, due to vasospasm, can lead to transmural ischemia with temporary ST elevation (**Fig. 61**).

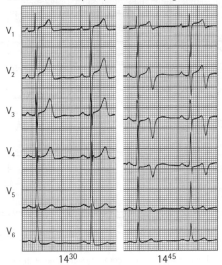

Fig. 61 Prinzmetal (variant) angina.

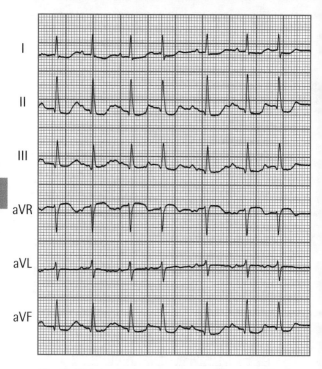

Fig. 62 ST depression in acute coronary syndrome with sinus tachycardia. The fourth beat shows a premature atrial contraction. An ST depression of up to 0.3 mV can be seen in V_4-V_6.

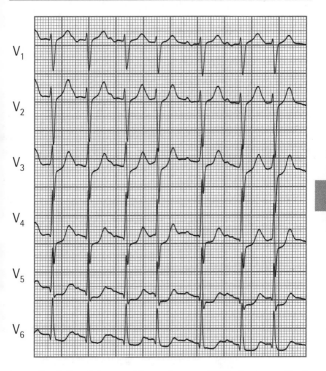

Resolution of the complaints and a normal ECG after two puffs of Glyceryl trinitrate.

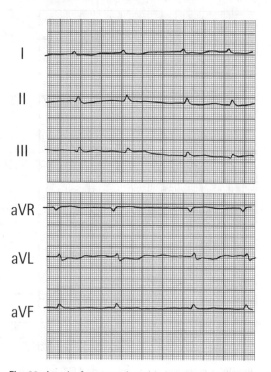

Fig. 63 Attack of acute angina with descending ST depression in V_3 and V_4.

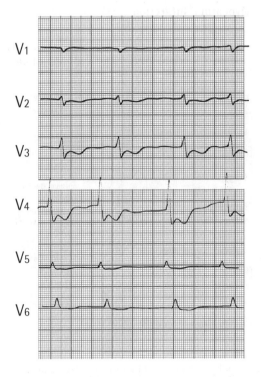

6.2 Myocardial Infarction

Definition
A myocardial infarction is transmural ischemia caused by the occlusion of a coronary artery and followed by typical sequential ECG changes (**Fig. 64**).

Stage	Age	ECG	Criteria
early stage	> a few minutes		high T waves
stage I	up to 6 hours		ST elevation R preserved no/small Q wave
intermed. stage	> 6 hours		ST elevation with T wave inversion loss of R wave, infarct Q
stage II	days		infarct Q T wave inversion ST normalization
stage III	residual		persistant Q loss of R wave T normalization

Fig. 64 Stages of myocardial infarction.

ECG
The **early stage** with a tall T wave is rarely seen, lasting only for a few minutes.

In **stage I**, ST elevation and R waves are present, there are no Q waves, and positive T waves can still be recorded. At this time the cardiac enzymes CK and CK-MB are usually not yet elevated and recanalization should be considered (thrombolysis or primary PTCA).

In the **intermediate stage** the ST elevation and the R amplitude decrease, Q waves arise and inverted T waves appear.

During the **next stage** the Q waves develop; the R wave will disappear.

In an old infarction (stage III) there is R wave loss in the anterior leads corresponding to the extent of the infarction.

Q waves may be found across the anterior myocardial wall, the T wave becomes positive again and the ST elevation disappears. Persistent ST elevations with inverted T waves are an indication of a ventricular aneurysm.

In **stage III** of a **posterior myocardial infarction,** significantly widened Q waves are found (**Fig. 65**) in leads II, III and aVF. Possible causes of Q waves are listed in **Fig. 66**.

In stage III of a posterior myocardial infarction, sometimes all ECG changes turn back to normal, so the infarction will be electrocardiographically silent. In this case the diagnosis has to be made by echocardiography showing irregular movement of the ventricles, by a ventriculography or by a scintiscan showing a perfusion deficit.

Localization

The area of ischemia is determined by the presence of ischemic changes in the corresponding ECG leads (**Fig. 58**).

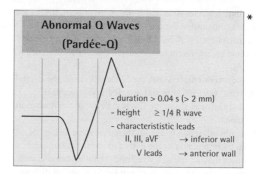

Fig. 65 Definition of infarction-related Q waves.

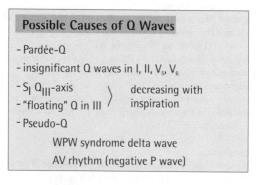

Fig. 66 Possible causes of Q waves.

ST depression in the reciprocal leads strongly suggests an acute myocardial infarction (**Fig. 67**). ST elevation on the anterior wall is accompanied by ST depression on the posterior wall and vice versa. These ECG changes in the reciprocal leads resolve within hours of infarction.

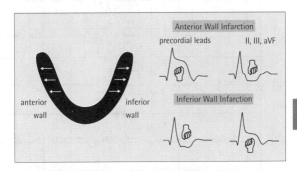

Fig. 67 Acute myocardial infarction: reflecting and reciprocal leads. Elevations over the anterior wall are accompanied by reciprocal depressions over the posterior wall.

The most important differential diagnoses
Acute pericarditis (p. 217)
Anterior subendocardial myocardial infarction (non-Q-wave infarction, p. 115)
Hypertrophic (obstructive) cardiomyopathy (p. 227)
Severe left ventricular hypertrophy (p. 38)

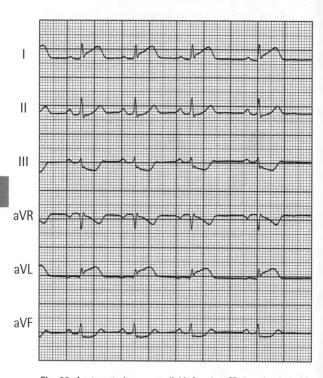

Fig. 68 Acute anterior myocardial infarction. ST elevation in I, aVL and V_1-V_4 accompanied by ST depression in II, III, aVF and V_6

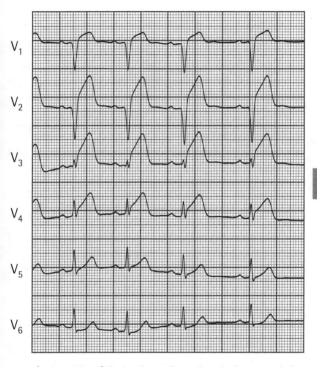

(reciprocal leads). During the cardiac catheterization, an occlusion of the left anterior descending artery was diagnosed.

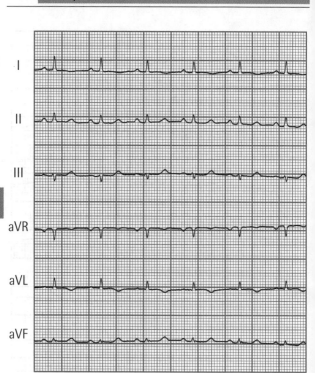

Fig. 69 Acute anterior myocardial infarction in the intermediate stage showing Q waves, a decrease in ST elevation and inversion

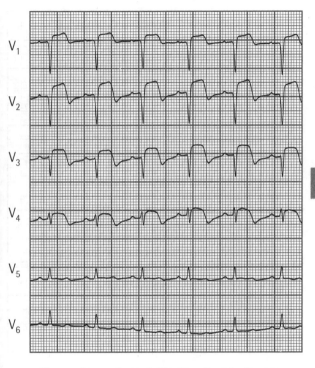

of T waves. Same patient as in **Fig. 68** on the following day.

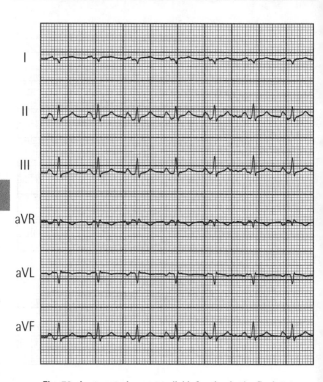

Fig. 70 Acute anterior myocardial infarction in the final state with a loss of the R waves in the anterior precordial leads.

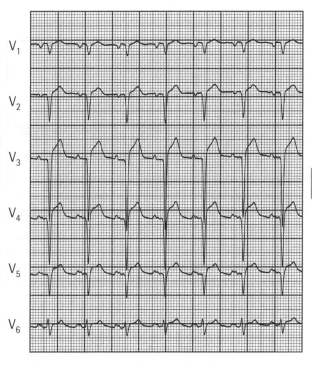

Again same patient as in **Fig. 68** and **Fig. 69**.

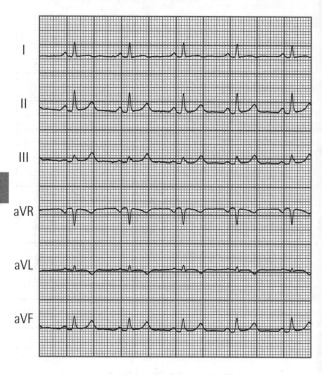

Fig. 71 Acute anterior myocardial infarction in the intermediate stage. R loss in the anterior precordial leads, deep Q waves,

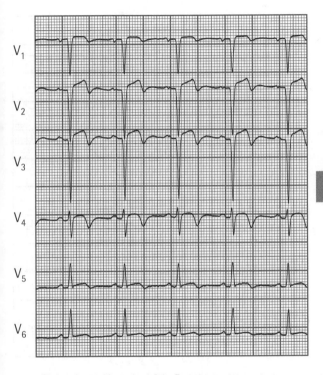

ST elevation and inversion of the T waves.

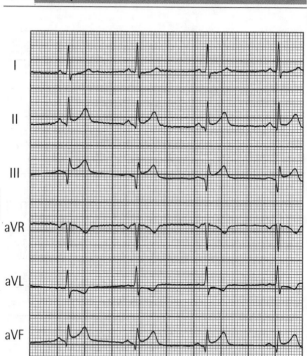

Fig. 72 Acute posterior myocardial infarction in stage I.
ST elevation in II, III and aVF. The T waves are still positive.

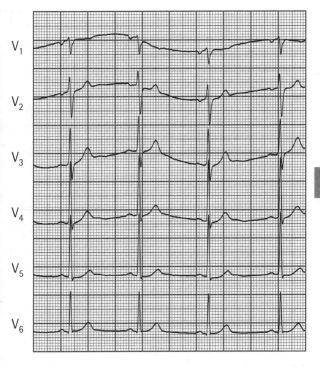

The Q waves in these leads indicate a former posterior myocardial infarction, stage III.

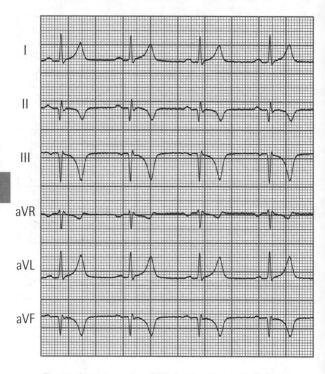

Fig. 73 Posterior myocardial infarction in stage II. After a drop in the ST elevation, Q waves and inverted T waves can be seen

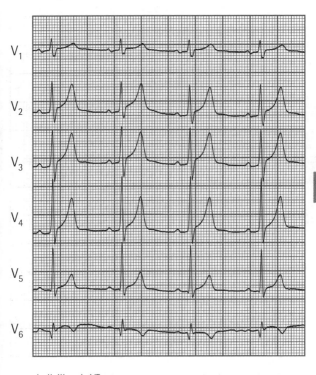

in II, III and aVF.

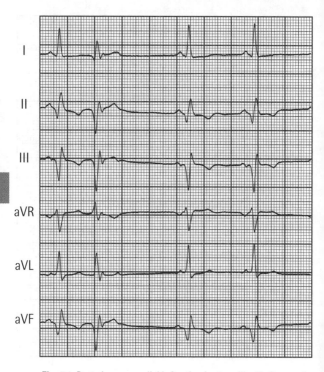

Fig. 74 Posterior myocardial infarction in stage III with Q waves in II, III and aVF.

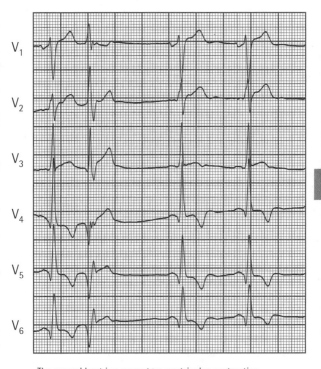

The second beat is a premature ventricular contraction.

6.3 Non-Q-Wave Myocardial Infarction

Definition
Subendocardial infarction of the anterior wall. A special form of the acute anterior myocardial infarction.

ECG
T wave inversion over the anterior precordial leads, without ST elevations, R loss or Q waves.

Prognosis
The prognosis of this form of MI does not differ significantly from that of a transmural anterior myocardial infarction.

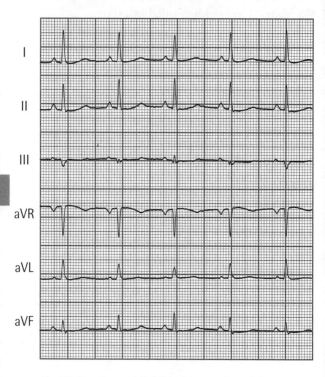

Fig. 75 Non-Q-wave infarction of the anterior wall. T wave inversion over the anterior leads, no ST elevation and normal

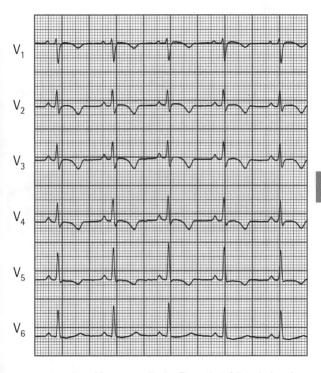

progression of R wave amplitudes. The patient felt typical angina.
The cardiac enzymes were elevated.

6.4 Stress Testing

Definition
Assessment of exercise related hypoperfusion of the heart.

Standardized exercise protocol
In order to obtain a high diagnostic value, the patient must undergo **maximum tolerable exercise**. This is defined by the age-adjusted values for max. heart rate (200 - age) and max. workload (watt) found in the standardized table.
If myocardial infarction happened recently a submaximal symptom-limited protocol should be used.

Age	Max. Heart Rate (min^{-1})	85% of max. Heart Rate (min^{-1})	Max. Work Men, 1.73 m^2 Body Surface (Watt)	Max. Work Women, 1.73 m^2 Body Surface (Watt)
20–29	195	170	170	140
30–39	189	160	140	120
40–49	182	150	110	110
50–59	170	140	100	90
60–69	162	130	80	80
70–80	145	120	50	50

The protocol should be adapted to the diagnostic goal. For the evaluation of coronary artery disease, increasing the exercise in three steps with each step lasting three minutes has proven effective to reach the max. age-adjusted workload (watt). Longer phases of exercise are useful for endurance testing.

Diagnostic value

Ascending ST depressions also occur in healthy people during vigorous exercise and tachycardia.

ECG criteria of myocardial ischemia are summarized in **Fig. 78**. Most common are horizontal and descending ST depressions (**Fig. 59**).

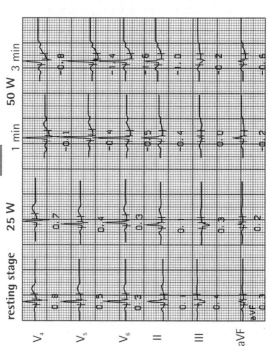

Fig. 76 Stress Test with CAD. Progressive ST depressions.

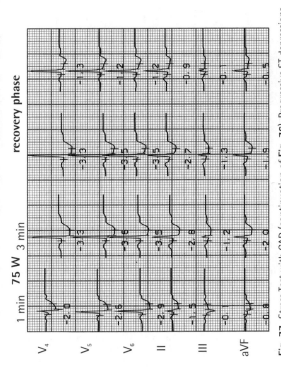

Fig. 77 Stress Test with CAD (continuation of **Fig. 76**). Progressive ST depressions, first horizontal, then descending.

**Stress Test
Predictors of CAD**

- horizontal or downsloping ST depression
  ≥ 0.2 mV
- upsloping ST depression, if
  J Point + 80 ms: ≥ 0.1 mV depressed
- ST elevation in leads
  without significant Q waves
- stress-induced typical angina
- stress-induced arrhythmia

Fig. 78 Stress Test: Predictors of CAD.

Indication

The diagnostic value of the exercise tolerance test depends on the prevalence of CAD in the tested sample. The higher the prevalence, the higher the predictive accuracy of the exercise tolerance test (Baye's theorem). It has not been shown beneficial to screen asymptomatic patients since the prevalence of CAD in this collective is too small. In women the accuracy of an exercise tolerance test is reduced due to a lower prevalence of CAD and a higher rate of false positive ECG changes showing typical horizontal or descending ST depressions. Cardiac catheterization of these patients is frequently normal. The classical indication for an exercise tolerance test with the highest predictive accuracy is **atypical chest pain in men > 40 years**. In case of typical chest pain/angina, cardiac catheterization is indicated even if the ECG is normal.

Complications
Although complications are rare during an exercise tolerance test, the criteria for stopping the test (**Fig. 79**) and contraindications (**Fig. 80**) must be observed.

Stop Criteria with Stress Testing

- progressive severe angina
- ST depression (horiz. or downsloping) $\geq$ 0.2 mV
- ST elevation in non-infarct related leads
- lack of increase, or decrease of blood pressure
- systolic blood pressure > 250 mmHg,
  diastolic blood pressure > 130 mmHg
- severe arrhythmics

Fig. 79 Stop criteria with stress testing.

Contraindications of Stress Testing

- unstable angina

- MI < 2 weeks

- critical aortic stenosis

- untreated hypertension

  if systolic value > 220 mmHg
  and/or diastolic value > 120 mmHg

- acute myocarditis or pericarditis

- decompensated heart failure

- severe arrhythmics

- thrombembolic conditions

Fig. 80 Contraindications of stress testing.

7. Bradyarrhythmias

7.1 Escape Rhythms

Pathophysiology

If the SA node fails to depolarize or the conduction of the depolarization wave is blocked, the pacemaker function will be taken over by a secondary site with a lower intrinsic frequency of depolarization than the SA node.

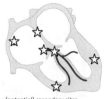

(potential) secondary sites

These slow rhythms originating from a secondary depolarization site are called "escape rhythms".

Forms

If the SA node fails to depolarize, control will be assumed by the **AV node** ("junctional escape rhythm"), which has a depolarization rate of 40-60 beats/min (p. 128). A third degree AV block can lead to an **escape rhythm** originating from the **bundle of His**. Although depolarization originates from this ventricular site, the QRS complex is not widened (**Fig. 54**, p. 83).

Fig. 56 (p. 86) shows a **ventricular escape rhythm** with a third degree AV block with broad QRS complexes and bradycardia.

Fig. 81 shows an **atrial escape rhythm**.

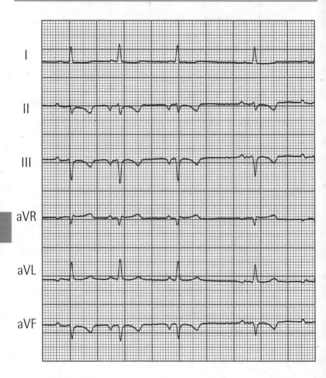

Fig. 81 Atrial escape rhythm, negative P waves in II and III. The fourth complex is a sinus beat with a positive P wave in II and III.

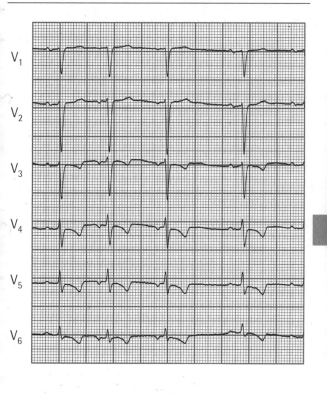

7.2 Junctional Escape Rhythms

Pathophysiology

If the SA node fails, an escape rhythm originating from the AV node can take over. The AV node can also initiate depolarization in healthy people without cardiac disease, for example, while

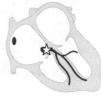

AV node rhythm

sleeping. Sometimes there is a "parasystolic rhythm" (simultaneous depolarization from two different sites with almost the same frequency). When this occurs, the sinus rhythm can convert into a junctional rhythm (AV node rhythm) and vice versa (AV dissociation). Treatment is not necessary.

The junctional escape rhythms are subdivided (Fig. 82)

1. Upper junctional rhythm

The atria are depolarized from the upper part of the AV node, therefore the P waves in I, II, III and aVF are negative. The PR interval can be shortened.

2. Central junctional rhythm

The depolarization site is in the middle of the AV node. Therefore, the atria and ventricles are depolarized at the same time and the P waves are hidden in the QRS complex (**Fig. 83**).

3. Lower junctional rhythm

The depolarization site is in the lower AV node close to the bundle of His. The atria are depolarized after the ventricles, and the P wave is located directly behind the QRS complex.

P waves are negative in I, II and III because of the retrograde depolarization (**Fig. 84**).

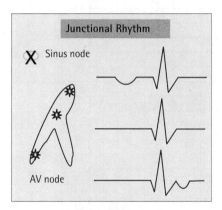

Fig. 82 Junctional rhythms. When originating in the **upper** AV node, P waves are negative and precede the QRS complex (PR may be shortened). If the origin is in the **middle parts** of the AV node, the P wave is absent (hidden in the QRS complex). **Lower** junctions are characterized by negative P waves following the QRS complex.

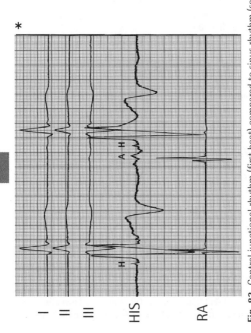

Fig. 83 Central junctional rhythm (first beat) compared to sinus rhythm (second beat). The atrial wave of the first beat, recorded in the right atrium (= RA) is located within the QRS complex. In the His ECG the A-wave cannot be identified. In sinus rhythm (second beat) the A-wave is regularly located before the QRS complex.

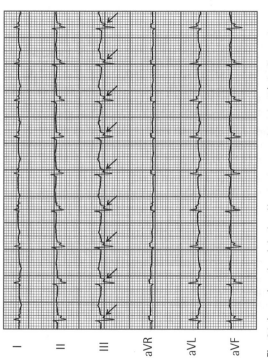

Fig. 84 Lower junctional rhythm. Heart rate approximately 45/min. P wave is detectable at the end of QRS in the ST segment. Paper speed is 12.5 mm/s.

7.3 Sinoatrial Block

Definition

Sinoatrial block is characterized
by the failure of the SA node
or a conduction defect between
the SA node and the atria, resulting
in a loss of atrial depolarization.
There is sinus arrest until an
escape mechanism takes over.

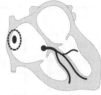

SA block

First degree sinoatrial block

Prolongation of the sinoatrial conduction time (not visible on a
standard ECG).

Second degree sinoatrial block,
type I, Wenckebach

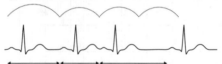

Progressive prolongation of the sinoatrial conduction with an
ultimate interruption in conduction.
PR intervals are constant while sinus intervals (PP interval) shorten
until a break occurs which is shorter than two PP intervals.

Second degree sinoatrial block, type II, Mobitz

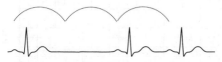

Intermittent sinus pauses that are a multiple of the sinus interval. A 2:1 block cannot be distinguished from a sinus bradycardia.

Third degree sinoatrial block

Complete block of the sinoatrial conduction with cardiac arrest and escape rhythm from a junctional or ventricular depolarization site.

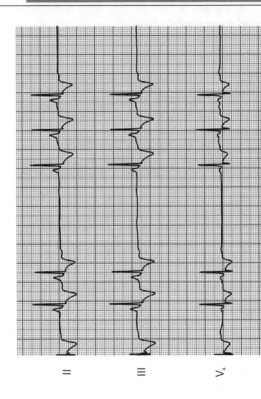

II

III

V₄

Fig. 85 Sinoatrial block. Sinus pauses without atrial depolarization (P waves).

7.4 Reflex Bradycardia

Clinical picture

Reflex bradycardia can lead to syncope.

Cardiac Syncopes

- Reflex mediated syncope
  - neurocardiogenic syncope
  - hypersensitive carotid sinus syndrome
  - reflex syncope associated with
    micturition / swallowing / coughing / pain /
    defecation

- Orthostatic syncope
- Arrhythmogenic syncope
- Mechanical obstructive syncope
  aortic stenosis, myxoma, pericordial tamponade,
  pulmonary emboli . . .

Fig. 86 Classification of cardiac syncopes.

1. Carotid sinus syndrome

Definition

Stimulation of a hypersensitive carotid sinus leads to bradycardia, including sinus arrest and hypotension.

Pathophysiology

The reflex pathway of the carotid sinus syndrome is shown in **Fig. 87**. Pressure on the carotid sinus or spontaneous turning of the head can cause sinus bradycardia and AV blocks, including third degree blocks, by a reflex activation of the vagal nerve. Vasodilation leading to hypotension can also be seen. Diagnostic criteria for carotid sinus syndrome are only fulfilled if the sinus arrest lasts longer than 6 seconds and the clinical symptoms like dizziness or syncope are triggered by a typical stimulus, for example syncope after sharply turning the head.

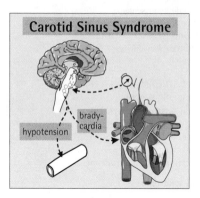

Fig. 87 Afferent impulses from the carotid glomus cause bradycardia and vasodilation by reflex activation of the vagal nerve.

Diagnosis

In a patient with a suspected hypersensitive carotid sinus, the carotid sinus should only be massaged when the patient is supine, a physician is present, IV access is available and atropine and adrenaline are at hand.

Carotid sinus massage

The carotid sinus massage (**Fig. 88**) is also indicated for the diagnosis of supraventricular tachycardia (see also p. 158). In this case there is no danger of symptomatic bradycardia (**Fig. 89**).

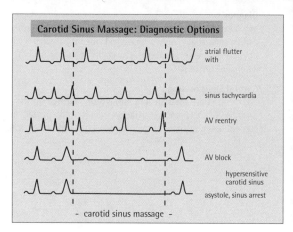

Fig. 88 Carotid sinus massage, diagnostic options.
In a regular sinus rhythm the carotid sinus massage can be used to diagnose a carotid sinus syndrome (caution: potentially dangerous). In supraventricular tachycardia it can be used to diagnose atrial flutter or to treat AV tachycardia and WPW tachycardia.

Treatment
In the case of marked reflex vasodilation, the implantation of a pacemaker is often ineffective!

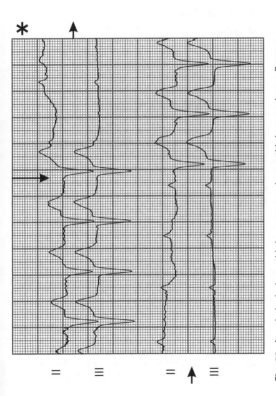

Fig. 89 A pathological carotid sinus massage in carotid sinus syndrome. Pressure on the carotid sinus results in AV block with a pause of 4.8 s and presyncope.

2. Neurocardiogenic Syncope

Pathophysiology

The neurocardiogenic syncope is caused by the stimulation of mechanoreceptors in the left ventricle (**Fig. 90**). It also results in bradycardia and peripheral vasodilatation leading to hypotension.

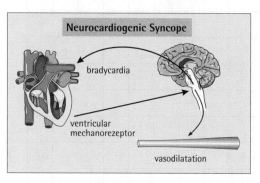

Neurocardiogenic Syncope

bradycardia

ventricular mechanorezeptor

vasodilatation

Fig. 90 Neurocardiogenic syncope. Stimulation of ventricular mechanoreceptors causes a reflex response with bradycardia and hypotension.

Diagnosis

A tilt test is useful in making a diagnosis. After a longer period in an upright position, sometimes syncope can be provoked by isoprenaline 1-5 mg/ min (**Fig. 91**) or nitroglycerin sublingually.

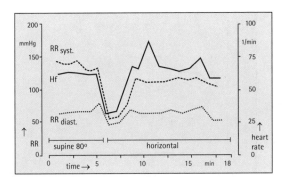

Fig. 91 Tilt table test with isoproterenol 2 mcg/min. After 5 min in supine position the patient feels dizziness and presyncope. Heart rate, systolic and diastolic blood pressure drop simultaneously. Symptoms disappear quickly, when the patient returns to horizontal position.

Treatment

Frequently the implantation of a pacemaker remains ineffective; syncopal episodes persist. Betablockers are the drug of choice (!), because their negative inotropic effect limits the hypersensitive mechanoreceptors (**Fig. 92**). Alternatively, disopyramide can be used for its negative inotropic effect.

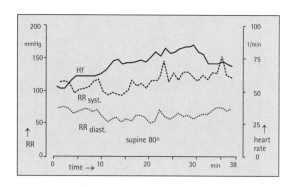

Fig. 92 Tilt table test with isoproterenol 4 mcg/min. After pretreatment with a betablocker the neurocardiogenic response is blunted (same patient as in **Fig. 91**).

7.5 Atrial Fibrillation with Bradycardia

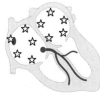

Definition
Atrial frequency of > 300/min with absolute arrhythmia and a ventricular rate of < 40 beats/min (bradycardia)
It is also called slow atrial fibrillation or atrial fibrillation with slow ventricular response.
(see also: atrial fibrillation with fast ventricular response, p. 150).

Atrial fibrillation

ECG

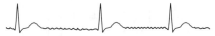

Absence of P waves, an irregular isoelectric line with bradycardia (< 40 beats /min) and absolute arrhythmia.

Cause
Most common in severe cardiac disease or sick sinus syndrome (p. 182).

Treatment
Before a pacemaker is considered, all drugs delaying the atrioventricular conduction (betablockers, calcium channel blockers of verapamil type, digoxin) have to be stopped. Proposed interventions in **Fig. 96**.

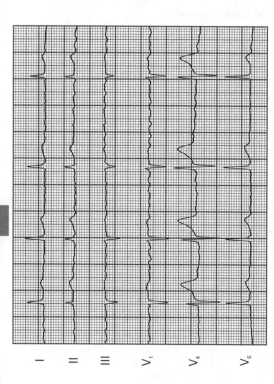

Fig. 93 Atrial fibrillation with slow ventricular response. Note an absolute arrhythmia as well as fine fibrillations, especially in V_1. Most commonly present in severe heart disease.

8. Tachyarrhythmias

8.1 General Description

Forms

Tachyarrhythmias include supraventricular (SVT) and ventricular tachycardias (VT).

Supraventricular tachycardias are characterized by a narrow QRS complex (< 0.12 s). The QRS complex is wide, however, if the SVT is associated with a bundle branch block.
A closer differentiation can be made by the position of the P wave in regards to the QRS complex (**Fig. 94**).

Ventricular tachycardias always have a widened QRS complex (> 0.12 s), except for the rare case in which it originates from the bundle of His.

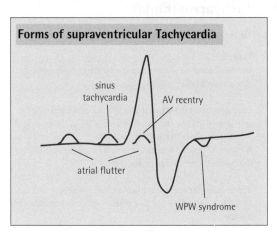

Fig. 94 Forms of supraventricular tachycardia, differentiated by the position of the P wave.

8.2 Sinus Tachycardia

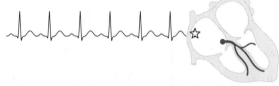

Supraventricular tachycardia

Definition
Supraventricular tachycardia with a frequency > 90 beats/min.

Causes
Primary sinus tachycardia, in some cases caused by a SA nodal reentry mechanism.
Secondary: hyperthyroidism, hypovolemia, heart failure and due to drugs, for example theophylline, catecholamines and reflex tachycardia during nifedipine therapy.

Treatment
Rare, primary sinus tachycardia can be treated with betablockers. In severe, intractable cases of SA node reentry an ablation in the area of the SA node has proven successful. In secondary sinus tachycardia, the underlying disease has to be treated.

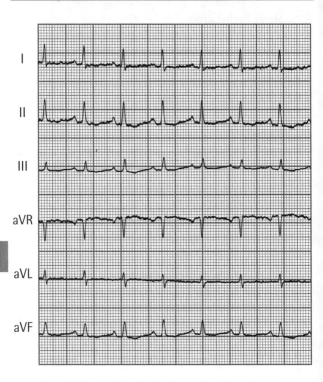

Fig. 95 Sinus tachycardia. The P wave is positive in leads I, II and III.

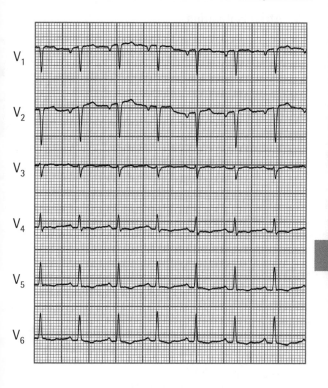

8.3 Atrial Fibrillation

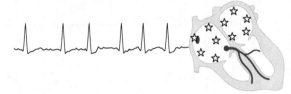

Definition
Atrial frequency of > 300/min with absolute arrhythmia and a
ventricular rate of > 90 beats/min
(see also atrial fibrillation with slow ventricular response, p. 143).

ECG
Absence of P waves, irregular isoelectric line.
The QRS complexes are usually narrow (**Fig. 100**).
If a wide QRS complex is present, the following differential
diagnoses have to be considered:
- existing bundle branch block
- aberrant conduction through the AV node
- atrial fibrillation in a WPW syndrome (p. 168).
Caution: Aberrant conduction with broad ventricular complexes is
often misinterpreted as ventricular runs. Sometimes atrial
fibrillation waves are easy, and sometimes very hard, to diagnose.
The irregular rate of the ventricular complexes help make the
diagnosis.

Treatment
A protocol is demonstrated in **Fig. 96**.

1. Heart rate control

In "fast" atrial fibrillation, rate control is most important. This is accomplished by digitalis, calcium channel blockers (verapamil) and betablockers. Both digitalis and calcium channel blockers are contraindicated for WPW syndrome with atrial fibrillation (**Fig. 111**, p. 177).

2. Anticoagulation

According to the textbooks, patients with atrial fibrillation existing for more than three days should be anticoagulated with heparin or warfarin for three weeks before attempting conversion. In some cases (**Fig. 97**), a transesophageal echocardiography (TEE), providing a high quality picture of the atria, is suitable for excluding a left atrial thrombus so that cardioversion may be performed immediately.

After successful cardioversion, anticoagulation therapy must be continued for 4 - 6 weeks, since atrial contraction is still compromised despite the sinus rhythm. If conversion to a sinus rhythm remains unsuccessful, long-term anticoagulation therapy is necessary (**Fig. 98**). Patients with a high embolic risk receive high dose warfarin, while those with a smaller risk with heart disease receive low dose warfarin therapy or 300 mg of aspirin a day. Idiopathic atrial fibrillation ("lone atrial fibrillation") with a normal left atrium does not require anticoagulation in patients < 60 years, while 300 mg of aspirin/day are recommended for older patients.

3. Contraindications for cardioversion

In patients with a severe underlying cardiac disease (status post myocardial infarction, severe congestive cardiomyopathy, severe mitral valve disease), cardioversion should only be attempted in individual cases. The success rate is low and the danger of provoking new arrhythmias is high (provocation of arrhythmias, p. 206). Patients with long-standing atrial fibrillation (> 12 months) or a severely enlarged atrium have a high recurrence rate.

4. Conversion

When indicated, conversion to sinus rhythm can be attempted by electrical cardioversion or by administering class I or class III antiarrhythmic.

After cardioversion, antiarrhythmics are often necessary in order to prevent relapses.

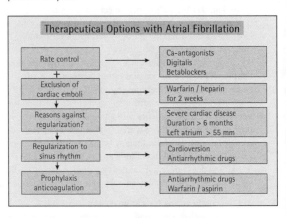

Fig. 96 Therapeutic options with atrial fibrillation.

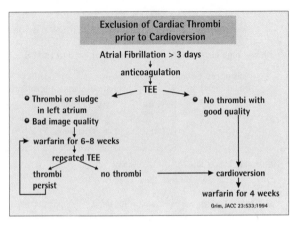

Fig. 97 Exclusion of cardiac thrombi prior to cardioversion.

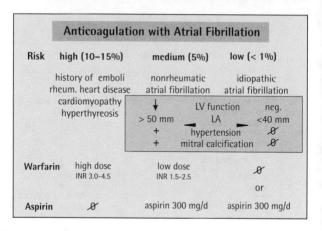

Fig. 98 Anticoagulation with chronic atrial fibrillation.

Precautions for Ambulatory Conversion of Atrial Fibrillation

exclusion of high risk patients

- No class I antiarrhythmics with CAD
- Avoid high doses of antiarrhythmic drugs and diuretics
- Control serum electrolytes, prophylactic substitution of K^+, Mg^{2+}
- Daily ECG
- Long-term ECG after 1–2 weeks
- Sufficient anticoagulation

Fig. 99 Precautions for ambulatory conversion of atrial fibrillation.

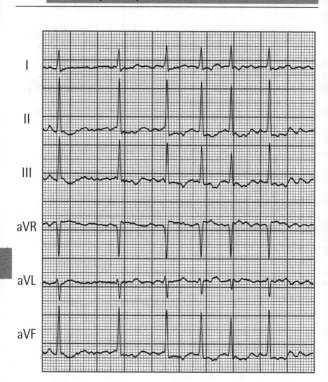

Fig. 100 Tachycardic atrial fibrillation with absolute arrhythmia. The mean heart rate is > 90/min.

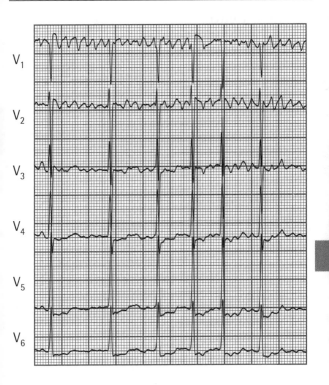

8.4 Atrial Flutter

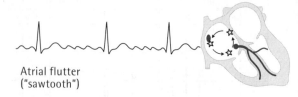

Atrial flutter
("sawtooth")

Definition
Atrial frequency of 240-300 beats/min.

ECG
Sawtooth-like P waves with regular or irregular ventricular conduction through the AV node. A 2:1 conduction may be mistaken for a sinus tachycardia (**Fig. 101**).

Diagnosis
In the case of a 2:1 conduction, a carotid sinus massage may be helpful in making the diagnosis (**Fig. 102**, also p. 137). Due to the delayed ventricular conduction, the sawtooth-like pattern of the P waves becomes evident. If a carotid sinus massage remains ineffective, adenosine 6-12 mg IV can be administered as a diagnostic test (**Fig. 103**).

Treatment
First line treatment is the same as in atrial fibrillation.

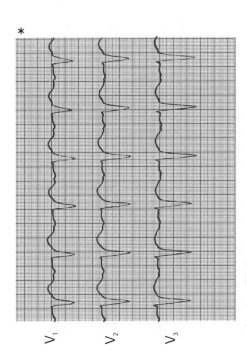

*

V₁

V₂

V₃

Fig. 101 Atrial flutter with 2 :1 conduction. Remark the P waves in the middle between two QRS complexes.

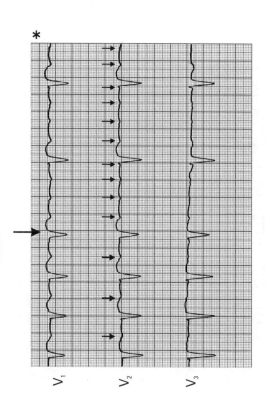

Fig. 102 Carotid sinus massage in atrial flutter (big arrow); the AV conduction is slowed down and additional P waves can be seen (small arrows).

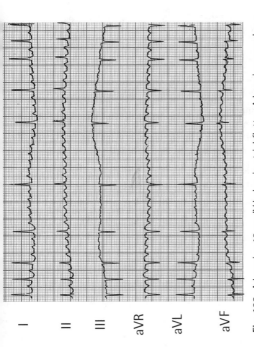

I

II

III

aVR

aVL

aVF

Fig. 103 Adenosine 12 mg IV bolus in atrial flutter. Adenosine provokes a temporary AV block, during which the sawtooth-like P waves become more evident. After 10 s, the rhythm returns to a regular tachycardia.

8.5 AV Nodal Reentry Tachycardia

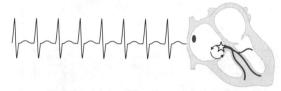

Definition

Reentrant tachycardia arising from the AV-node.

Epidemiology

Common form of supraventricular tachycardia, most common cause of paroxysmal supraventricular tachycardia (PSVT) more common in women.

Pathophysiology

A tachycardia occurs when an impulse deviates into a circular conduction pathway, forming a loop. In typical AV reentry, the impulse runs through a slow pathway first and backwards through a fast pathway in the AV node. In an atypical AV reentry, the depolarization wave runs the other way around (**Fig. 104**).

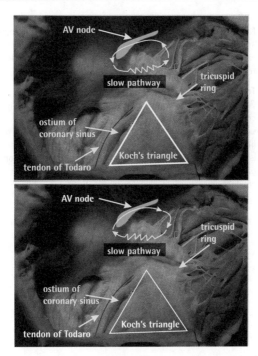

Fig. 104 AV nodal reentry tachycardia. In typical forms (top) there is a counterclockwise reentry with retrograde passage through the AV node. In atypical cases the reentry runs clockwise.

ECG

Narrow QRS complexes. The P waves are hidden in the QRS complex and are usually not visible in a standard ECG (sometimes in the early ST segment and the QRS complex). An AV reentry can lead to repolarization disturbances and ST depression.

Treatment

Good response to verapamil and adenosine IV. If the AV reentry is chronic, vagal maneuvers such as a carotid sinus massage or swallowing ice water can be attempted. If still unsuccessful, drugs like verapamil or antiarrhythmics can be used. Curative treatment is possible through a catheter ablation of the slow conduction pathway (pacemaker only necessary in rare cases) or the fast conduction pathway (pacemaker frequently necessary).

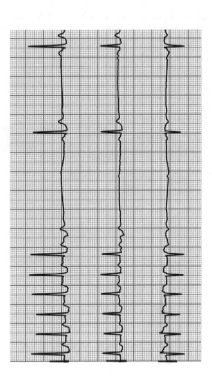

Fig. 105 Interruption of an AV nodal reentry tachycardia with an IV bolus of 12 mg adenosine. Within a few seconds the supraventricular tachycardia (narrow QRS complexes without P waves) converts to a sinus rhythm.

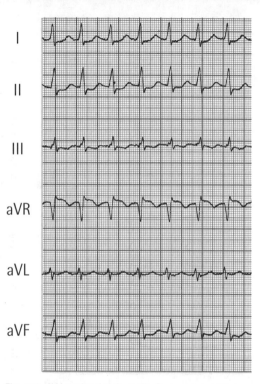

Fig. 106 AV junctional tachycardia. P waves not visible. ST depression in V_2-V_6 due to tachycardia.

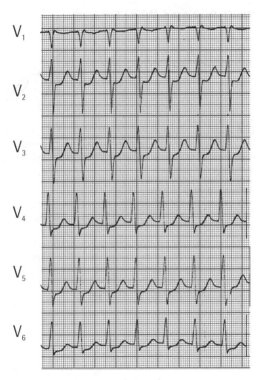

The QRS complex is narrow (< 0.12 s).

8.6 Wolff-Parkinson-White Syndrome

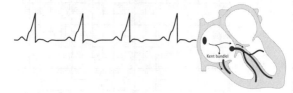

Definition

The WPW syndrome is a congenital syndrome with premature depolarization (preexcitation) of the ventricles through accessory AV conduction pathways.

Pathophysiology

An accessory muscular bundle, the Kent bundle, conducts the electrical impulse from the atria to the ventricles. Depolarization through the Kent bundle reaches the ventricles faster than the one leading through the AV node or the bundle of His, so that some parts of the ventricle get depolarized earlier than others stimulated by the normal conduction pathway. The two different conduction pathways between atria and ventricles can lead to various arrhythmias. These are shown in **Fig. 107**.

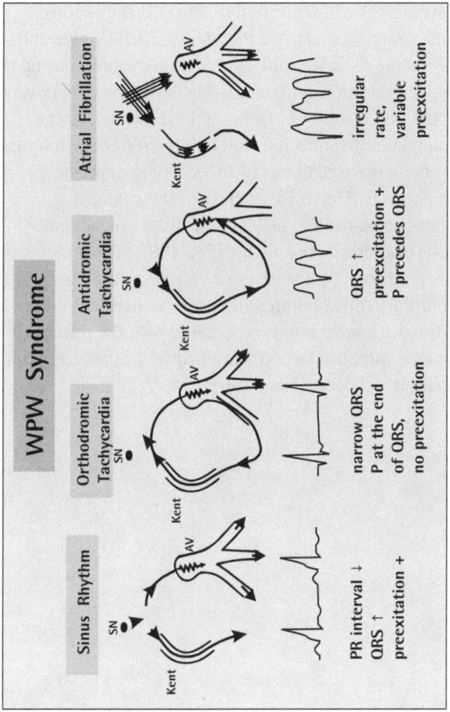

Fig. 107 Forms of arrhythmias with WPW syndrome. Preexcitation is always present, if antegrade conduction occurs from the atrium to the ventricle via the accessory pathway.

ECG

In a WPW syndrome with sinus rhythm, the ECG shows three characteristic changes: shortened PR intervals, delta waves and widened QRS complexes. The initial aberrant activation causing the ventricular depolarization generates a slurring of the QRS, or wave. The rest of the QRS complex has a normal pattern due to the regular completion of conduction through the AV node. In sinus rhythm, the delta wave can be used to localize the accessory conduction pathway (**Fig. 108**). Because of the changed depolarization, repolarization may also be disturbed, adding repolarization disorders to the picture (**Fig. 109**). In general, a delta wave occurs if an anterograde accessory conduction pathway from the atrium to the ventricle is present. In the "concealed" WPW syndrome, the delta wave is missing because only the retrograde conduction runs through the accessory pathway. Supraventricular tachycardias can still occur (**Fig. 110**).

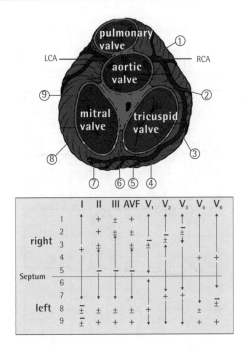

Fig. 108 Localization of the accessory pathway on the basis of preexcitation in the surface ECG.

+ means positive orientation of the preexcitation,

- means negative orientation of the preexcitation.

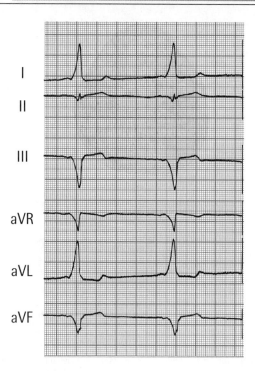

Fig. 109 WPW syndrome with sinus rhythm. The PR interval is shortened, the QRS complex widened (> 0.12s) with an obvious delta wave and repolarization disturbances caused by the

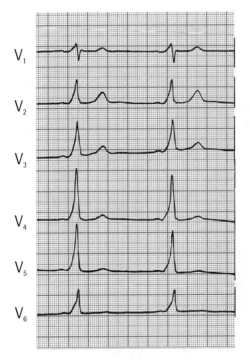

accessory conduction pathway. Negative delta waves in III and aVF can look like a Q wave in a posterior myocardial infarction (paper speed of 50 mm/s).

*

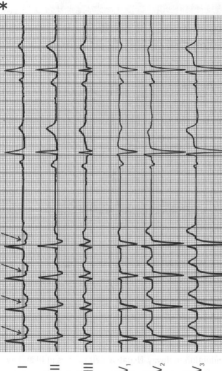

I

II

III

V₁

V₂

V₃

Fig. 110 Orthodromic tachycardia in a WPW syndrome during the transition to sinus rhythm. During the tachycardia, the QRS complex is narrow; the P wave can be found at the end of the QRS complex. Interruption of the tachycardia with adenosine 12 mg IV. During sinus rhythm no delta waves can be seen (concealed WPW syndrome).

In a WPW syndrome the following arrhythmias can occur (also **Fig. 107**):

1. Orthodromic tachycardias

There is a circular conduction pathway with an anterograde depolarization via the AV node and retrograde conduction via the accessory conduction pathway (**Fig. 110**). The tachycardias are regular with a narrow ventricular complex, and the P waves are situated at the end of the QRS complex in the early ST segment. During the tachycardia, delta waves are not present. Sometimes a rate-induced intermittent BBB occurs. If the ventricular rate slows down, the accessory pathway is located on the same site as the BBB (in a RBBB on the right hand side).

2. Antidromic tachycardia

In this case, the circular conduction pathway is reversed: antegrade depolarization of the ventricles via the accessory pathway and retrograde depolarization via the AV node. Only approx. 15% of all WPW tachycardias are antidromic. The ECG shows a delta wave, a short PR interval and broad QRS complexes.

3. Atrial fibrillation in a WPW syndrome

Due to competitive conduction to the ventricle between the AV node and an accessory pathway, an absolute arrhythmia results (variable RR intervals) showing a delta wave of changing morphology (variable QRS complexes, **Fig. 111**). AF is the most serious form of an arrhythmia in a WPW syndrome because it can induce ventricular fibrillation. Drugs that interfere with AV conduction, like calcium channel blockers, digitalis or adenosine, are contraindicated (**Fig. 112**).

Fig. 113 provides a summary of preexcitation syndromes.

Treatment

Asymptomatic patients with WPW syndrome do not require treatment.

In many patients, **tachycardias** can be suppressed for years by vagal stimulation: drinking ice water, carotid sinus massage, intraabdominal pressure, or forced swallowing.

Orthodromic tachycardias can be treated with betablockers, calcium channel blockers (verapamil type) and in an acute situation with adenosine IV. These drugs lead to an interruption of the circular conduction in the AV node (**Fig. 114**).

Atrial fibrillation with anterograde activation of the accessory pathway can be treated with class I or class III antiarrhythmics. These lead to a blockage of the accessory pathway.

In recurrent **paroxysmal palpitations**, a radiofrequency catheter ablation of the accessory conduction pathway is indicated. This is particularly effective in drug-resistant cases, in patients wishing to become pregnant (due to the danger of an aggravation of the arrhythmias and contraindications for antiarrhythmic drugs during pregnancy) and also in recorded atrial fibrillation in a WPW syndrome.

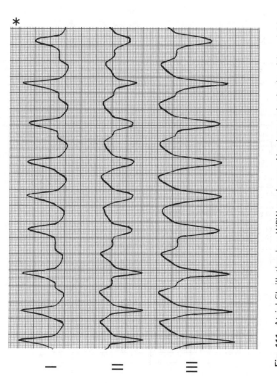

*

— = ≡

Fig. 111 Atrial fibrillation in a WPW syndrome. Absolute arrhythmia with variable RR intervals and variable QRS complex morphology.

*

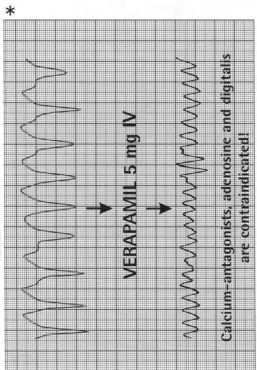

VERAPAMIL 5 mg IV

Calcium-antagonists, adenosine and digitalis are contraindicated!

Fig. 112 Induction of ventricular fibrillation after administration of Verapamil 5 mg IV in a case of WPW syndrome and atrial fibrillation. The AV conduction is slowed down with calcium channel blockers, digitalis and adenosine, with simultaneous faster conduction in the accessory pathway.

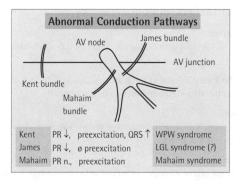

Fig. 113 Forms of arrhythmia due to abnormal conduction.

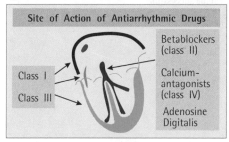

Fig. 114 Site of action of antiarrhythmic drugs. Betablockers, calcium-antagonists, adenosine and digitalis work on the AV node. Class I and III antiarrhythmic drugs work on the atrial and ventricular muscle and accessory pathways.

8.7 Atrial Tachycardia

Definition
Atrial tachycardia with P waves at a rate of 100 - 200/min.

ECG
Regular P waves, some of them are negative in II, III and aVF. It frequently has variable conduction to the ventricles.

Etiology
Often there is an underlying cardiac disease like pulmonary hypertension or heart failure.

Treatment
Verapamil can be effective, otherwise other antiarrhythmic drugs are indicated. Also, a radiofrequency catheter ablation of the atrial focus can be successful.

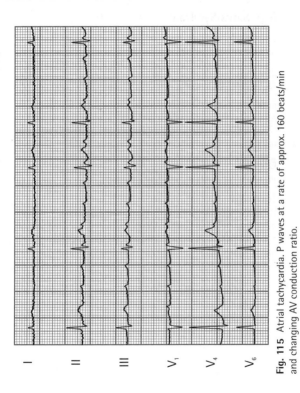

I

II

III

V₁

V₄

V₆

Fig. 115 Atrial tachycardia. P waves at a rate of approx. 160 beats/min and changing AV conduction ratio.

8.8 Sick Sinus Syndrome

Definition
Supraventricular arrhythmias due to sinus node dysfunction.

Synonym
Tachycardia-bradycardia syndrome ("tachy-brady" syndrome)

ECG
Alternating tachycardic (atrial fibrillation, atrial flutter, atrial tachycardias) and bradycardic arrhythmias (sinoatrial block, sinus bradycardia). Sometimes an AV block occurs.

Etiology
Inflammation, arteriosclerosis or ischemia.

Treatment
Often the therapy consists of a pacemaker implantation in order to be able to treat tachycardic episodes with negative chronotropic drugs (betablockers, calcium channel blockers, digitalis, antiarrhythmics).

8.9 Premature Atrial Contractions (PACs)

Definition
Premature atrial beats caused by an ectopic (non-sinus) focus within the atria.

ECG
Ectopic beats with a non-widened QRS complex which are nearly identical to a sinus induced QRS, frequently preceded by an abnormal P wave. PACs can alter the sinus cadence and also occur in runs.

Treatment
As most patients are not hemodynamically compromised, no treatment is necessary. Hyperthyroidism should be excluded. In severe cases, betablockers are indicated.

Premature Atrial Contractions (PACs) 185

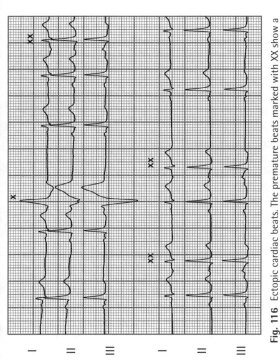

Fig. 116 Ectopic cardiac beats. The premature beats marked with XX show a narrow QRS complex and are nearly identical to the sinus induced QRS complexes. → PACs. (X) Premature ventricular contraction with a broad QRS.

8.10 Premature Ventricular Contractions (PVCs)

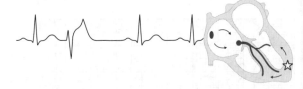

Definition
Premature ventricular depolarization arising from an ectopic focus in the ventricles.

ECG/pathophysiology
Extra beats with a broad (> 0.12 s) and bizarre QRS complex. Uniformly shaped (monomorphic) ectopic beats lead to the conclusion that they are of unifocal origin (monotope). Multiform (polymorphic) ectopic beats result from a multifocal origin.

PVCs lead to a compensatory pause if they displace the sinus node activity by retrograde conduction through the AV node, otherwise they are interpolated between two normal beats.

In **bigeminy** every sinus beat is followed by a ventricular premature beat (**Fig. 119**); in **trigeminy** every sinus beat is followed by two PVCs. Ectopic beats may occur as **couples**, **runs** or continuously, leading to persistent ventricular tachycardia (**Fig. 120**). In the **R on T phenomenon**, PVCs fall simultaneously with the upstroke or peak of the T wave of the previous beat.

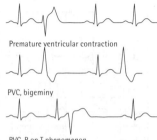

Premature ventricular contraction

PVC, bigeminy

PVC, R on T phenomenon

Lown classification of PVCs

This widespread grading system is controversial since a rise in the grade does not necessarily mean an increase in severity. For example, severe multiform PVCs (Class III) are certainly more hemodynamically relevant and dangerous than a single ventricular couplet (Class IVa).

Grade	Description
Grade 0	no PVCs
Grade I	occasional unifocal PVCs (< 30/h)
Grade II	frequent unifocal PVCs (> 30/h)
Grade III	multiform PVCs
Grade IVa	couplets (two consecutive PVCs)
Grade IVb	runs (repetitive PVCs of 3 or more) or ventricular tachycardia
Grade V	early PVCs (R on T phenomenon)

Fig. 117 Lown classification.

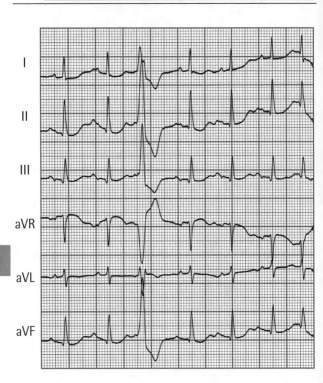

Fig. 118 PVCs. The ectopic beat has a BBB-like shape followed by a compensatory pause.

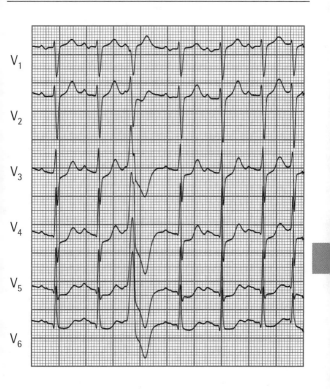

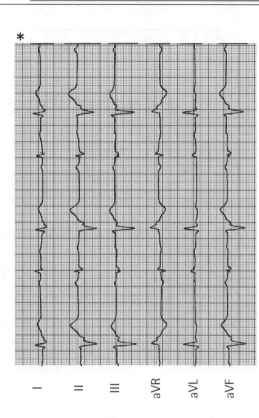

Fig. 119 Bigeminy. Every normal QRS is followed by a PVC.

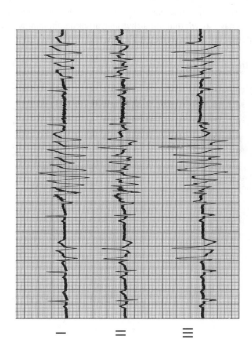

Fig. 120 Run of PVCs. On the left is a couplet, followed by a multifocal run. The patient was asymptomatic following myocardial infarction.

Treatment

With underlying cardiac disease, frequent PVCs indicate a higher risk of sustained ventricular tachycardia or fibrillation. However, studies have shown that antiarrhythmic drugs do not improve the prognosis, but rather worsen it (CAST study).

The treatment is demonstrated in **Fig. 121**.

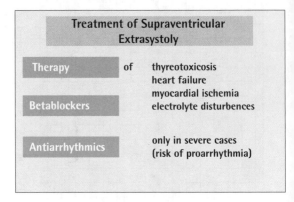

Fig. 121 Treatment of PVC (and PAC).

8.11 Sustained Ventricular Tachycardia

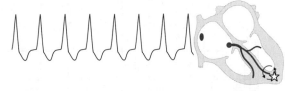

Definition
Tachycardia originating from a ventricular focus and lasting > 30 s.

ECG
Broad QRS complexes at a rate of > 90 beats/min.
The ventricular ectopic beats can be of a single morphology
(uniform ventricular tachycardia, **Fig. 122, Fig. 123**), of different
morphologies (multiform ventricular tachycardias) or of changing
polarity (torsade de pointes, frequently induced by antiarrhythmic
drugs).

Caution
Ventricular tachycardias are always a life threatening complication
and require observation and treatment in a coronary care unit!

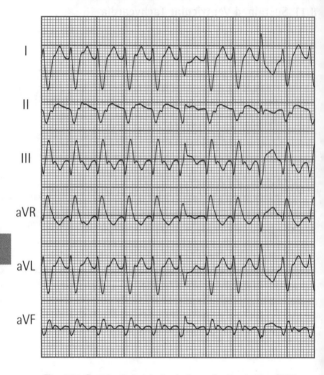

Fig. 122 Sustained ventricular tachycardia. Heart rate of 150 beats/min, the QRS complexes are wide and have a RBBB-like

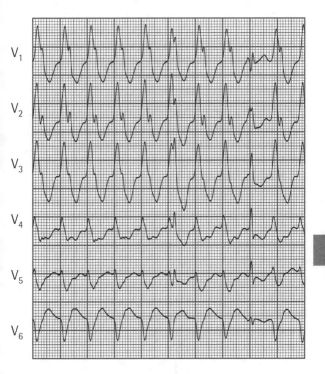

shape due to the ectopic focus in the left ventricle.

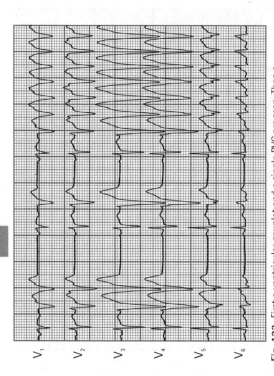

Fig. 123 First a ventricular couplet and a single PVC are seen. Then a sustained uniform ventricular tachycardia with a LBBB-like picture (focus in the right ventricle) begins.

Treatment

Emergency guidelines are shown in **Fig. 126**.

For diagnostic purposes and initiating antiarrhythmic treatment, a programmed ventricular stimulation is helpful. Here, the heart is stimulated by an electric catheter situated in the right ventricle (**Fig. 124**).

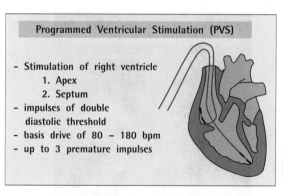

Programmed Ventricular Stimulation (PVS)

- Stimulation of right ventricle
    1. Apex
    2. Septum
- impulses of double diastolic threshold
- basis drive of 80 – 180 bpm
- up to 3 premature impulses

Fig. 124 Programmed ventricular stimulation (PVS)

A basic stimulation (S_1) is followed by premature impulses (S_2, S_3, S_4) that may induce a ventricular tachycardia (**Fig. 127**). This tachycardia can then be interrupted by a ventricular overdrive stimulation (**Fig. 128**) or must be cardioverted. Afterwards the patient is treated with antiarrhythmic drugs for several days and the programmed ventricular stimulation is repeated. Once the induction of ventricular tachycardias has ceased, the patient has a good long-term prognosis. If the ventricular tachycardia is still inducible, the implantation of an automatic cardioverter defibrillator (ICD) should be considered (**Fig. 125**). An ICD monitors the heart rhythm, recognizes sustained ventricular tachycardias and automatically delivers a ventricular overdrive stimulation. If these measures remain ineffective, the heart is shocked.

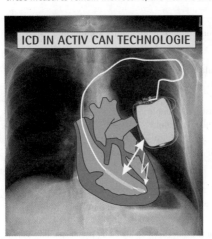

Fig. 125 Implantable cardioverter defibrillator (ICD). This special pacemaker monitors the heart rhythm and delivers an electroshock from the pacemaker to the electrode if ventricular tachycardia or fibrillation is registered (Active Can technology).

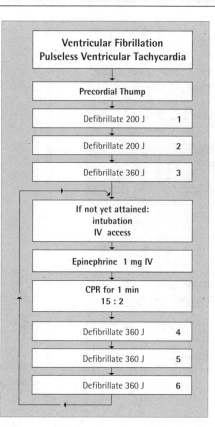

Fig. 126 Emergency guidelines in ventricular tachycardia/fibrillation. All efforts to restore the normal rhythm must comply with the guidelines of general resuscitation.

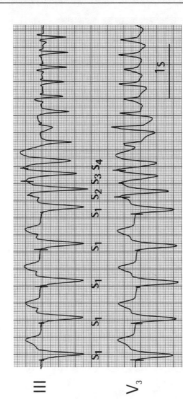

Fig. 127 Induction of a sustained ventricular tachycardia by ventricular stimulation. A basic stimulation (S_1) is followed by three premature impulses (S_2, S_3, S_4) inducing ventricular tachycardia.

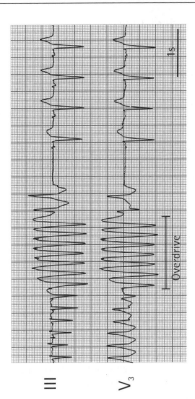

III

V$_3$

Fig. 128 Interruption of ventricular tachycardia by ventricular overdrive stimulation. Ventricular stimulation at a higher rate than the ventricular tachycardia (overdrive pacing) can interrupt tachycardia. This is associated with a potential risk of inducing ventricular fibrillation.

8.12 Ventricular Fibrillation

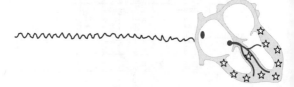

Definition
Chaotic ventricular electrical discharge from multiple reentry loops
resulting in hemodynamic collapse (**Fig. 129**). **Sudden cardiac
death**: unexpected death within 1 h after becoming symptomatic
(**Fig. 130**).

Cause
The most common cause of ventricular fibrillation (VF) is acute
ischemia resulting from myocardial infarction (**Fig. 129**). The most
common causes of sudden cardiac death are fast ventricular
tachycardias and ventricular fibrillation.

Prognosis
Patients who have survived episodes of ventricular fibrillation
should be treated in a coronary care unit even in the absence of
myocardial infarction. The predictive value of controlled ventricular
stimulation is less than in monomorphic tachycardias.

Treatment
In acute VF, emergency therapy is electrical defibrillation. In
chronic VF, an implantable automatic defibrillator may be
necessary (**Fig. 125**).

*

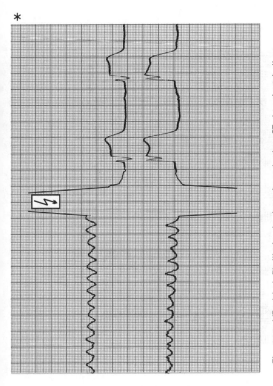

Fig. 129 VF with defibrillation back to sinus rhythm. ST elevations indicate an acute myocardial infarction causing the arrhythmia.

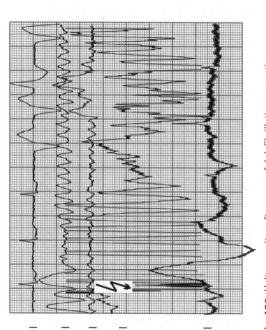

Fig. 130 Holter monitor after successful defibrillation preventing sudden cardiac death. A sinus rhythm converts to ventricular tachycardia which quickly degenerates to ventricular fibrillation.

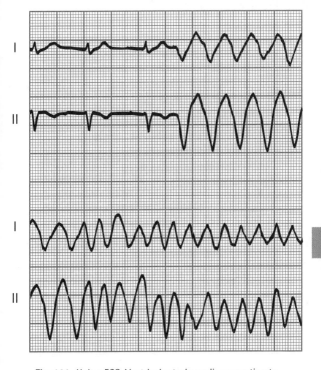

Fig. 131 Holter ECG. Ventricular tachycardia converting to ventricular fibrillation.

8.13 Proarrhythmia

Definition

Deterioration or primary occurrence of arrhythmias with antiarrhythmic drug therapy.

Forms

Forms of proarrhythmias are demonstrated in **Fig. 132**. torsade de pointes are characteristic and dangerous (**Fig. 133**).

They frequently arise from a bradycardia following an episode of a fast-slow-fast heart rate.

Proarrhythmia with Antiarrhythmic Drugs	
New demonstration of:	**Deterioration of preexistant arrhythmia**
• PVCs	• Increase of ectopic beats in Holter ECG from (PVC / h)
• Ventricular runs (repetitive PVCs)	
• Continuous VT	10 - 50 x 10
• Torsades de pointes	51 - 100 x 5
• Ventricular fibrillation	101 - 300 x 4
	> 300 x 3
	• Runs x 10
	• Incessant VT
	• Inability to terminate VT by cardioversion

Fig. 132 Definition and forms of proarrhythmia.

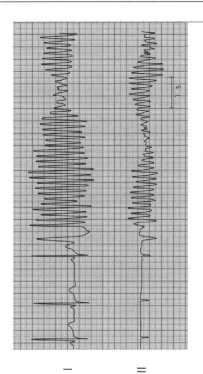

Fig. 133 Torsade de pointes secondary to antiarrhythmic treatment. A ventricular ectopic beat triggers a multiform ventricular tachycardia with changing polarization of the QRS complex.

Predisposition

Predisposing is a secondary "long QT syndrome" with prolongation of the heart-rate-dependent QT interval (**Fig. 134, Fig. 135**, also long QT syndrome, p. 214, **Fig. 139**).

Prevention

All antiarrhythmic drugs may produce proarrhythmias and must be used with caution especially in outpatients.

The most important issue is the **exclusion of high risk patients** with a low probability of a conversion to a sinus rhythm, but a high risk of arrhythmias: mitral valve disease, severe coronary heart disease, severe congestive cardiomyopathy, a left atrium > 55 mm, duration of atrial fibrillation > 6 months.

A **holter monitor** should be performed 14 days after the start of antiarrhythmic drug therapy and also after every dose adjustment (**Fig. 136**).

High doses of antiarrhythmic drugs should be avoided, as well as the use of diuretics, which can contribute to electrolyte disturbances.

A daily ECG is necessary during the initial phase of therapy to determine the QTc (also **Fig. 99**, p. 155).

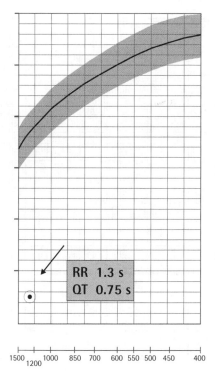

RR 1.3 s
QT 0.75 s

1500 1200 1000 850 700 600 550 500 450 400

Fig. 134 Corrected QT (QTc) used for the ECG in **Fig. 135**.

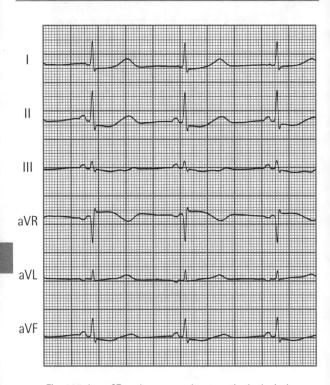

Fig. 135 Long QT syndrome secondary to antiarrhythmic drugs. The QT interval is 0.75 s, heart rate > 46 beats/min,

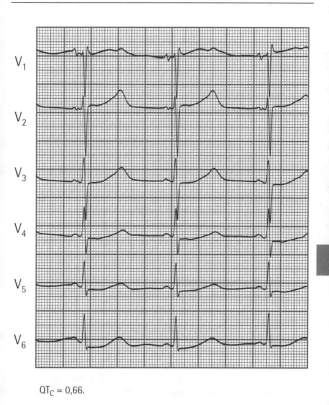

QT$_C$ = 0,66.

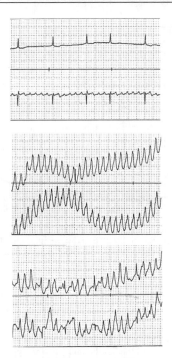

Fig. 136 Proarrhythmia with intermittent atrial flutter with flecainide therapy (100 mg three times daily). Holter monitor with atrial flutter, irregular conduction (top) and episodes of up to 10 s of ventricular flutter.

Treatment

Guidelines for acute therapy are shown in **Fig. 137**.

Proarrhythmia:

Treatment of Torsades de pointes

- NO Antiarrhythmica
- Magnesium infusion 1–2 g i.v.
- titrate K^+ to high levels (5 mM)
- refer to hospital
- temporary pacing at 100 bpm

Fig. 137 Proarrhythmia: treatment of torsades de pointes.

Magnesium Treatment of Torsades de Pointes

$MgSO_4$ 2 g Bolus / 2 min (≈16.2 mval)	
partial success	repeat after 10min
	2–10 mg / min $MgSO_4$
if ineffective	pacing at ~ 100 bpm
	isoproterenol 1 – 5 µg / min

Keren, Cardiovasc Drugs 1991; 5:509

Fig. 138 High dose magnesium therapy in case of torsades de pointes tachycardia. Although effective, the QT_C interval remains unchanged!

8.14 Long QT Syndrome

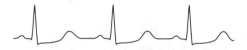

Definition
Abnormal prolongation of the corrected QT interval (QTc) predisposing to malignant cardiac arrhythmias (multiform ventricular tachycardia, torsade de pointes).

Etiology
The prolongation of the QT interval is a sign of repolarization disorders which predispose to arrhythmias.
Primary long QT syndromes are congenital (Jervell-Lange-Nielsen syndrome without deafness, Romano-Ward syndrome with deafness). A family history of sudden cardiac death and syncope is typical.
Secondary long QT syndromes occur with antiarrhythmic drug therapy, tricyclic antidepressants and some antibiotics, for example erythromycin. A prolongation of QTc > 0.46 s indicates a proarrhythmic risk (**Fig. 135**).

Diagnosis
The prolongation of the QT interval can be calculated using a nomogram or the Bazett's formula (**Fig. 139**).

Treatment
Primary long QT syndromes can be treated with high dose betablockers, by modification of the autonomic innervation of the

heart through surgical procedure or symptomatically with an implantable defibrillator.

Most importantly, in a secondary proarrhythmia, all causative agents must be discontinued. Also see proarrhythmia, p. 206.

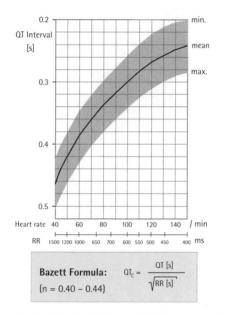

$$QT_c = \frac{QT\ [s]}{\sqrt{RR\ [s]}}$$

Bazett Formula:
(n = 0.40 – 0.44)

Fig. 139 Corrected QT interval (QTc): nomogram, Bazett´s formula.

9. Carditis, Cardiomyopathy

9.1 Acute Pericarditis

Pathophysiology
Inflammation of the pericardium can lead to subepicardial ischemia with ST elevations.

ECG
ST elevations, typically originating from the S wave. In certain cases, the ECG can be misinterpreted as a myocardial infarction (**Fig. 140**).

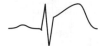

Diagnosis
Signs of pericarditis:
- absence of ST depressions in the reciprocal leads
- simultaneous ST elevations on the anterior and posterior wall
- ECG changes lasting for several days
- pericardial rub (not in an effusion)
- signs of inflammation (elevated CRP, elevated ESR, leukocytosis, fever)
- thoracic pains resistant to glyceryl trinitrate

The last three signs do not exclude a myocardial infarction (p. 96). If in doubt, a diagnostic cardiac catheterization may be necessary.

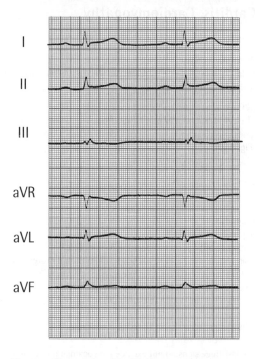

Fig. 140 Acute pericarditis. ST elevations in the leads over the anterior (I, V$_2$ - V$_6$) and posterior myocardial wall (II, aVF)

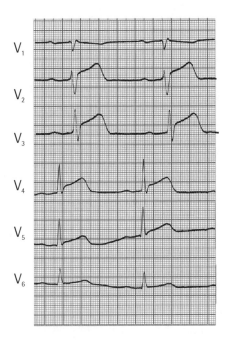

originating from the S wave.

9.2 Low Voltage QRS

Definition
Peripheral low voltage QRS: amplitude < 0.5 mV in the limb leads I, II and III (**Fig. 141**).
Central low voltage QRS: amplitude < 0.5 mV in I, II and III and < 0.7 mV in the precordial leads, **Fig. 142**).

Pathophysiology
Peripheral low voltage QRS: particularly in pulmonary emphysema, poor skin contact of the electrodes or obesity.
Central low voltage: caused by insulation in the area immediately surrounding the heart, indicating a pericardial effusion. A cardiac tamponade is not a diagnosis seen on an ECG, but a description of typical hemodynamic changes caused by a pericardial effusion and leading to cardiogenic shock (tachycardia, hypotension, high CVP with elevated jugular venous pressure).

Diagnosis
The echocardiography is the most useful study to diagnose a pericardial effusion.

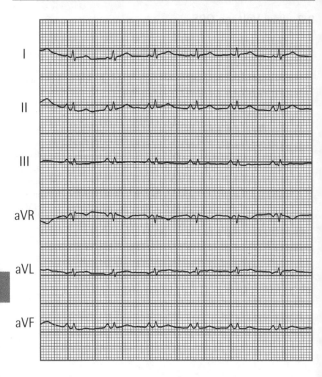

Fig. 141 Peripheral low voltage QRS. QRS amplitudes in the limb leads are < 0.5 mV, QRS amplitudes in the precordial leads

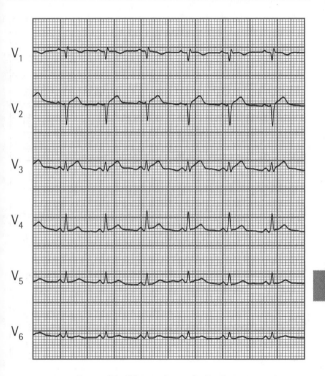

are normal caused, in this case, by marked pulmonary emphysema.

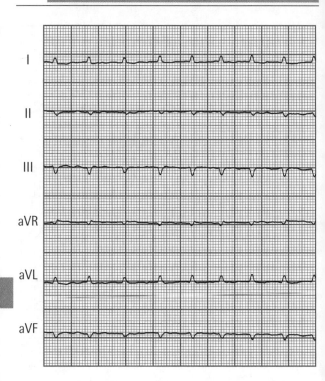

Fig. 142 Central low voltage QRS. The QRS amplitude is < 0.5 mV in the limb leads and < 0.7 mV in the precordial leads, caused

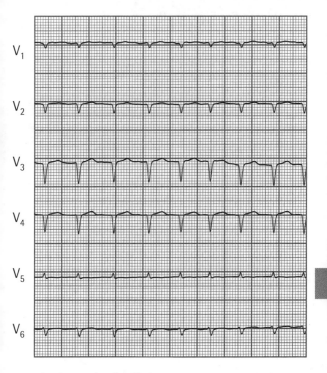

by a large pericardial effusion.

9.3 Dilated Cardiomyopathy

Definition
Progressive dilation of the left ventricle with thinning of the ventricular wall and the clinical features of cardiac failure.

Causes
Long-standing hypertension, chronic myocarditis, idiopathic dilated cardiomyopathy (DCM) and valvular heart disease with left ventricular overload, for example aortic regurgitation. A similar picture can be seen in ischemic cardiomyopathy due to severe coronary heart disease.

ECG
Dilated cardiomyopathy has no specific ECG signs. The ECG shows nonspecific repolarization disturbances, bundle branch like pictures and arrhythmias (PVCs, atrial fibrillation, **Fig. 143**).
In an ischemic cardiomyopathy, signs of one or several old myocardial infarctions (p. 96-p. 112) may be found.

Further diagnostic tests
An echocardiogram evaluates the size and shape of the heart and the ventricular function. To diagnose the underlying disease, a cardiac catheterization is often necessary.

9.4 Hypertrophic Cardiomyopathy

Definition

Hypertrophic obstructive cardiomyopathy: progressive myocardial hypertrophy, affecting primarily the left ventricle, resulting in reduced diastolic ventricular filling. A massively thickened interventricular septum can obstruct the left ventricular outflow pathway.

ECG

Signs of left ventricular hypertrophy (p. 38), varying ST segment changes (elevations and depressions) without classic localization and deep inverted T waves (s. **Fig. 144**).

Further diagnostic tests

Echocardiography (hypertrophic ventricular wall, thickened interventricular septum, subvalvular aortic stenosis in doppler ultrasound), cardiac catheterization, respiration dependent systolic murmur on auscultation.

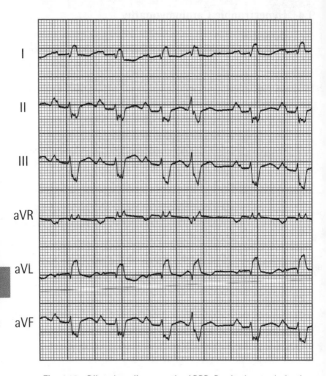

Fig. 143 Dilated cardiomyopathy. LBBB, P-mitrale, repolarization disorders caused by the LBBB.

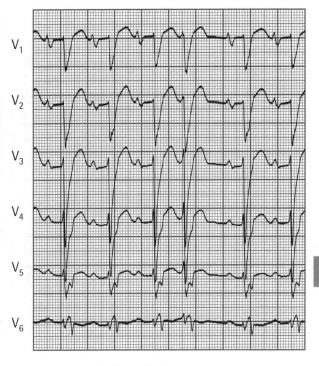

Premature ventricular contractions.

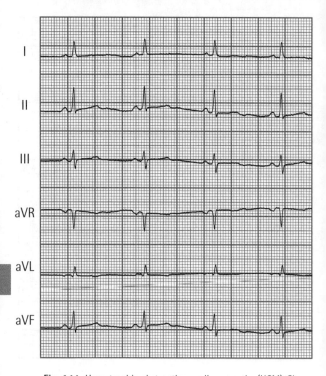

Fig. 144 Hypertrophic obstructive cardiomyopathy (HCM). Signs of left ventricular hypertrophy (S in V_2 + R in V_5 > 3.5 mV),

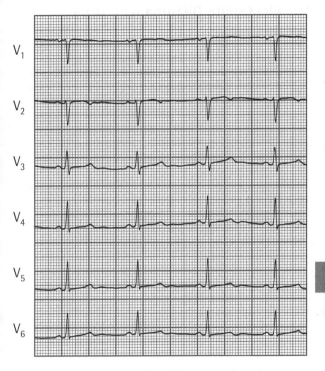

depression and elevation of the ST segment as signs of a
pseudoinfarction.

10. Electrolyte Disturbances, Drugs

10.1 Hypokalemia

Hypokalemia causes repolarization disorders, ST depressions and prominent U waves that may merge into TU waves. Hypokalemia predisposes to arrhythmias such as atrial fibrillation, ventricular fibrillation and PVCs.

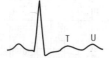

10.2 Hyperkalemia

Hyperkalemia initially appears with tall, peaked T waves that later flatten. A broad QRS complex appears. Finally, tachycardic arrhythmias can occur resulting in bradycardia and asystole.

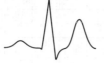

10.3 Hypercalcemia

Hypercalcemia leads to a shortening of the corrected QT interval (QTc) (normogram, **Fig. 10**, p. 17).

QT shortened

10.4 Hypocalcemia

Hypocalcemia leads to a prolongation of the QT interval.

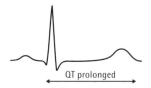

QT prolonged

Note
In all electrolyte disturbances, there is no exact correlation between ECG changes and the serum level.

10.5 ECG Changes induced by Digitalis

ECG

At therapeutic serum levels the ECG shows shallow ST depressions (**Fig. 145**).

Digitalis overdose presents arrhythmias like premature atrial beats and AV blocks (II°+ III°).

Caution

The effects of glycosides are increased by hypokalemia and hypercalcemia (p. 232, p. 232).

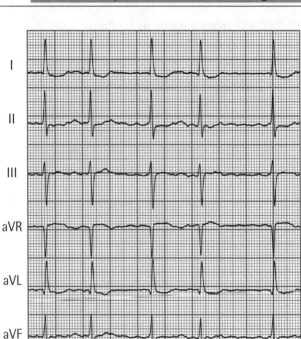

Fig. 145 Absolute arrhythmia in atrial fibrillation with digitalis therapy. The glycosides were given to control the patient's

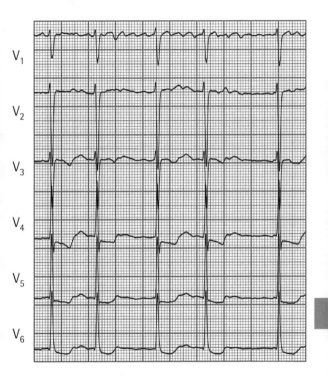

ventricular rate. Negative shallow ST depressions in V_5 and V_6.

10.6 Betablockers, Ca-Channel Blockers

Caution

The following drugs can cause a dose-dependent first degree AV block, in rare cases also II° and III° AV block:

- calcium channel blockers, like verapamil
- betablockers
- antiarrhythmic drugs with betablocking side effects (sotalol, propafenone)
- cardiac glycosides (p. 235).

Particularly in sick sinus syndrome, these drugs are contraindicated or must be administered with special caution. Before implanting a pacemaker, these drugs should be discontinued.

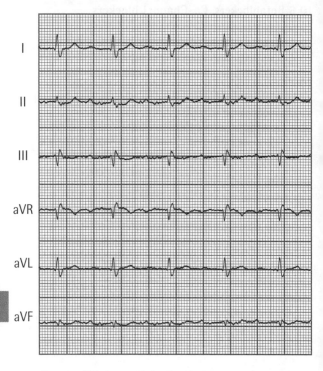

Fig. 146 ECG changes during betablocker therapy (metoprolol 100 mg twice daily). First degree AV block with an old RBBB.

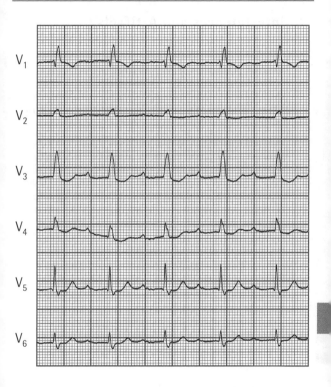

11. Interferences and Artifacts

11.1 Incorrect Polarization

Incorrect polarization of the limb leads
Incorrect polarization of the limb leads can be recognized by abnormal or non-existing axis deviations (for example negative QRS in I, II, III) and particularly in comparison to an old ECG (**Fig. 147**).

Incorrect polarization of the chest leads
Incorrect polarization of the chest leads can be recognized by an abnormal R progression from V_1-V_6. If the electrodes are placed too high (in the third or even second intercostal space), the ECG shows a diminished R progression or R loss over the anterior wall and may be incorrectly diagnosed as an old anterior myocardial infarction (**Fig. 148**).

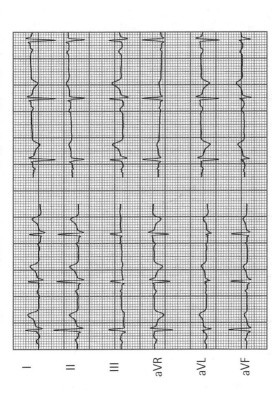

I

II

III

aVR

aVL

aVF

Fig. 147 Incorrect polarization in I shown on the right (yellow cable/right arm, red cable/left arm). Correct polarization is shown on the left.

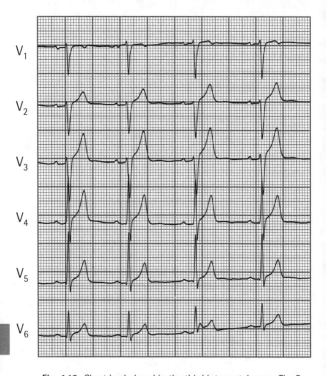

Fig. 148 Chest lead placed in the third intercostal space. The R amplitudes in V_1–V_3 are reduced, which may be mistaken for an

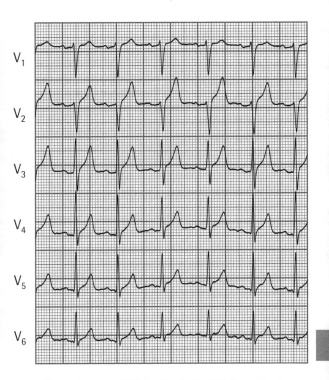

old anterior myocardial infarction (to the left). Correct lead positions on the right!

11.2 Further Disturbances and Artifacts

Mains noise

A frequent disturbance signal is mains noise (**Fig. 149**). This is easily detectable at the 50 Hz frequency. There is no physiological ECG signal at this high frequency. Possible causes are a missing grounding (black wire either missing or defect) or loops caused by contact between the metal cover and fingers or toes. In any case, correcting the underlying cause is preferred to inserting a filter. ECG machines frequently have a "notch filter" which selectively extracts oscillations of 50 Hz.

Muscular shivering

Muscular shivering is also irregular and in a high frequency range (**Fig. 150**). Often a P wave cannot be clearly identified and can be mistaken for atrial fibrillation (without absolute arrhythmia!). Causal relief is preferred (relaxed position, pillow under the knees, blanket for shivering)

Disconnected electrodes

Disconnected electrodes can lead to an incorrect diagnosis. Atrial fibrillation can be misdiagnosed in V_1 in **Fig. 151**. With a closer look, regular P waves can be seen in the other leads. The cause was a defect in a wire in lead V_1.

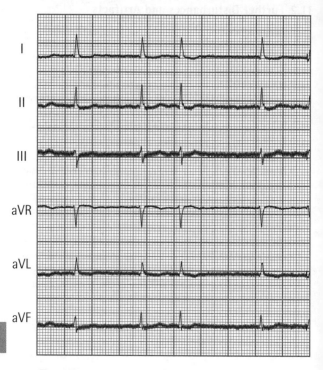

Fig. 149 Disturbances secondary to mains noise: high frequency disturbance at 50 Hz.

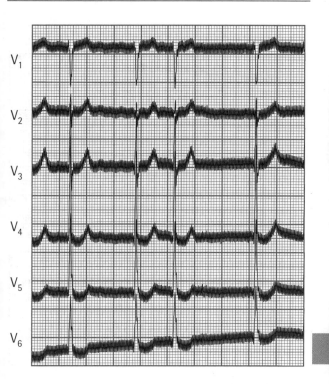

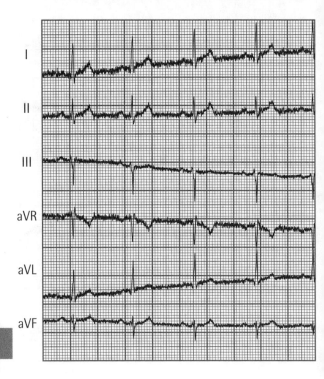

Fig. 150 Muscular shivering is also a high frequency disturbance with an irregular pattern.

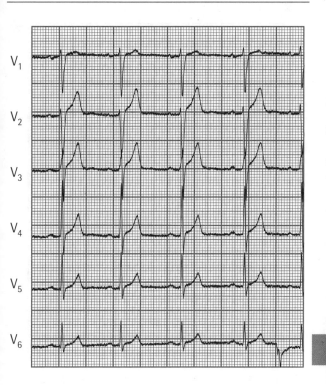

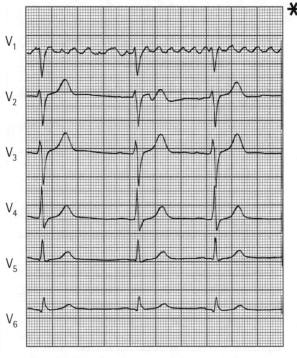

Fig. 151 Disconnected electrode in V_1. Atrial fibrillation can be incorrectly diagnosed, but there are regular P waves in the other leads.

Notes

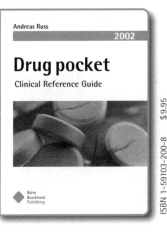
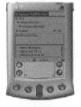

Create a set!

pocketcards cover medical information: pocket-sized, printed in color on white plastic.

Each **pocketcard** provides a practical summary of essential information about common aspects of everyday medical practice.

Antibiotics pocketcard 2002 ($3.95)
BLS/ALS pocketcard ($3.95)
ECG pocketcard ($3.95)
ECG Evaluation pocketcard ($3.95)
ECG Ruler pocketcard ($3.95)
ECG pocketcards ($9.95, set of 3 cards)
Emergency Drugs pocketcard ($3.95)
H&P pocketcard ($3.95)
Medical Abbreviations pocketcard ($6.95, 2 cards)
Medical Spanish pocketcard ($3.95)
Neurology pocketcard ($6.95, 2 cards)
Normal Values pocketcard ($3.95)

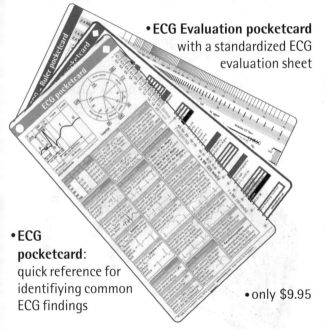

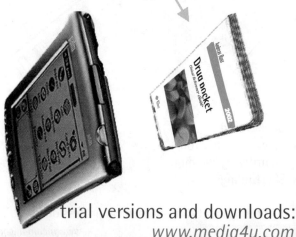

Medical Spanish pocket

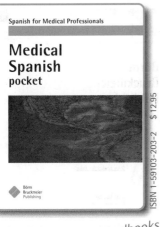

Spanish for Medical Professionals

Medical Spanish pocket

ISBN 1-59103-203-2

$ 12.95

Börm Bruckmeier Publishing

- vital communication tool for anyone working with Spanish-speaking patients
- clearly organized by situation: interview, examination, course of visit
- bilingual dictionary containing Spanish medical terminology specific to Mexico, Puerto Rico, Cuba and other countries
- provides hundreds of essential words and phrases, ready to use
- for residents and all other medical professionals

more pocket-sized handbooks

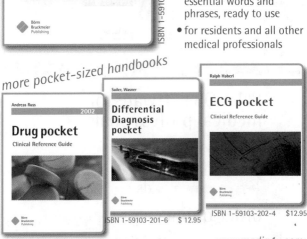

Andreas Russ

2002

Drug pocket

Clinical Reference Guide

Börm Bruckmeier Publishing

ISBN 1-59103-200-8 $9.95

Sailer, Wasner

Differential Diagnosis pocket

Börm Bruckmeier Publishing

ISBN 1-59103-201-6 $ 12.95

Ralph Haberl

ECG pocket

Clinical Reference Guide

Börm Bruckmeier Publishing

ISBN 1-59103-202-4 $12.95

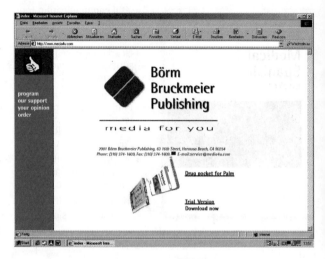

Palm OS software for
medical professionals

support
→ free updates
→ free downloads

order online

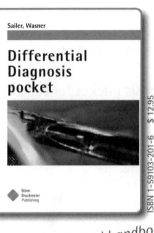
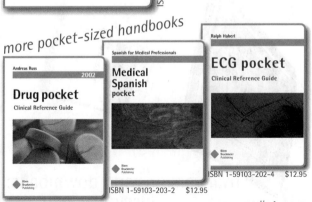

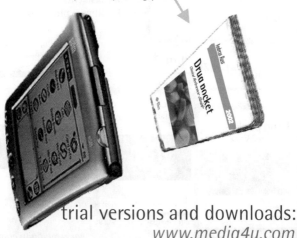

Index

Quick Reference

Hypertrophy of the Heart
Right Atrial Enlargement
P-pulmonale:
elevated, peaked P wave > 0.2 mV,
particularly in II, III and aVF.

Left Atrial Enlargement
P-mitrale:
widening of the P wave > 0.1 s,
particularly in I, II and $V_1 - V_3$.
In V_1 often a biphasic P wave with a
marked negative deflection.

Right Ventricular Hypertrophy
Sokolow index: R in V_2 + S in V_5
> 1.05 mV, normal axis/vertical range or
right axis deviation, sometimes RBBB-like
ECG.

Left Ventricular Hypertrophy
Sokolow-Index: S in V_2 + R in V_5
> 3,5 mV, normal axis/horizontal range -
left axis deviation.

Bundle Branch Blocks
Left Anterior Fascicular Block
No widening of the QRS, but left axis
deviation.

Left Posterior Fascicular Block
No widening of the QRS, but right axis
deviation.

Incomplete Left Bundle Branch Block
Widening of the QRS > 0.10 s,

but < 0.12 s, often R-reduction over the anterior wall.

Complete LBBB
Widening of the QRS > 0.12 s, delay of terminal deflection in V_6 > 0.05 s, frequently R-loss over the anterior wall, left precordial repolarization disturbances and ST-elevation.

Incomplete RBBB
Widening of the QRS complex > 0.10 s, but < 0.12 s, delay in terminal deflection of > 0.03 s in V_1, often R prime (R') in V_1.

Complete RBBB
Widening of the QRS > 0.12 s, delay in terminal deflection in V_1 > 0.03 s, frequently rSr' complex in V_1, repolarization disturbances in V_1–V_3.

AV Blocks

1° AV Block
Consistent delay in conduction, PQ interval > 0.20 s, every P wave is followed by a QRS complex.

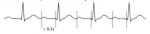

2° AV Block, Mobitz Type I (Wenckebach)
Intermittent conduction failure with missing QRS complexes, progressive prolongation of the PR interval until a P wave is blocked and the QRS complex is dropped.

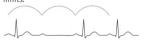

2° AV Block, Mobitz Type II
Intermittent failure of the AV conduction, the PR interval remains within normal limits.

3° AV Block (Complete Block)
Complete conduction block of all electrical impulses between atria and ventricles. Atria and ventricles beat

independently. Escape mechanism localized in the bundle of His (small QRS) or in the ventricle (BBB-like QRS).

Stage	Age	ECG	Criteria
early stage	> a few minutes		high T waves
stage I	up to 6 hours		ST elevation R preserved no/small Q wave
intermed. stage	> 6 hours		ST elevation with T wave inversion loss of R wave, infarct Q
stage II	days		infarct Q T wave inversion ST normalization
stage III	residual		persistant Q loss of R wave T normalization

Myocardial Ischemia
Angina
Horizontal or descending ST depression.

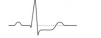

Myocardial Infarction
Early stage: Tall T wave.
Stage I: ST elevation and R waves are present, no Q waves, T waves are still positive.
Intermediate Stage: ST elevation and R wave decrease, Q waves arise and inverted T waves appear.
Next Stage: Q waves develop, R wave disappears.
Stage III: Loss of R wave in the anterior leads. Q waves may be found over the anterior myocardial wall, T wave becomes positive again and ST elevation disappears.

Non-Q-Wave Myocardial Infarction
Subendocardial infarction of the anterior wall with T wave inversion over the anterior wall, no ST elevations, no R loss and no development of Q waves.

Bradyarrhythmias
Junctional Escape Rhythms

1. Upper junctional rhythm:
P waves in I, II, III and aVF are negative,
PQ Interval can be short.

2. Central junctional rhythm:
P waves are hidden in the QRS

3. Lower junctional rhythm:
P waves are negative in I, II, III and
located behind QRS complex.

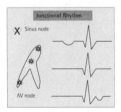

Sinoatrial Block

1° SA Block
Prolongation of the sinoatrial conduction
time. Not visible in standard ECG.

2° SA Block, Type I Wenckebach
Progressive prolongation of the SA
conduction with an ultimate interruption
in conduction. PR intervals are constant
while sinus intervals (PP interval) shorten
until a break occurs which is shorter than
two PP intervals.

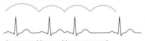

2° SA Block, Type II Mobitz
Intermittent sinus pauses that are a
multiple of the sinus interval.

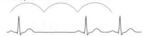

3° SA Block
Complete block. Cardiac arrest and escape
rhythm from a junctional or ventricular
depolarization site.

Reflex Bradycardia:
Carotid sinus syndrome

Pressure on the carotid sinus can cause sinus bradycardia and AV block. Vasodilatation leading to hypotension can be seen.

Neurocardiogenic Syncope

Caused by stimulation of mechanoreceptors in the left ventricle. It results in bradycardia and peripheral vasodilatation leading to hypotension.

Atrial Fibrillation with Bradycardia

Absence of P waves, an irregular isoelectric line with bradycardia and absolute arrhythmia.

Tachyarrhythmias
Sinus Tachycardia

Supraventricular tachycardia with a frequency of > 90 beats/min.

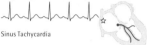

Sinus Tachycardia

Atrial Fibrillation

No P waves, irregular isoelectric line. Atrial frequency of > 300/min with absolute arrhythmia and a ventricular rate of > 90 beats/min.

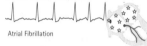

Atrial Fibrillation

Atrial Flutter

Atrial frequency of 240 - 300 beats/min, sawtooth-like P waves with regular or irregular ventricular conduction through the AV node.

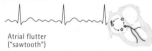

Atrial flutter
("sawtooth")

AV Nodal Reentry Tachycardia

Narrow QRS. P waves hidden in the QRS. AV reentry can lead to repolarization disturbances and ST depression.

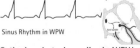

AV Nodal Reentry Tachycardia

WPW Syndrome
Sinus Rhythm in WPW:
Shortened PQ intervals, delta waves, QRS > 0.12 s, repolarization disturbances.

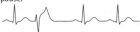

Sinus Rhythm in WPW

Orthodromic tachycardias in WPW
Regular tachycardia, narrow QRS complex, P waves at the end of QRS in the early ST segment, no Delta waves.

Antidromic tachycardia in WPW
Regular tachycardia, significant delta waves, short PQ interval, broad QRS complex.

Atrial Fibrillation in WPW
Variable RR intervals (absolute arrhythmia), delta wave of changing morphology (variable QRS complexes).

Atrial Tachycardia
Regular P waves with a rate of 100 - 200 beats/min. Some of the P waves are negative in II, III and aVF.

Sick Sinus Syndrome
Alternating tachycardic (atrial fibrillation, atrial flutter, atrial tachycardias) and bradycardic arrhythmias (sinoatrial block, sinus bradycardia), sometimes an AV block occurs.

Premature Ventricular Contractions (PVCs)
Extra beats with a broad (> 0.12 s) and bizarre QRS. Sometimes compensatory pause.

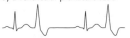

Bigeminus: Every sinus beat is followed by a ventricular premature beat.

Trigeminus: Every second sinus beat is followed by a PVC.

Couples, Runs

R-on-T-phenomenon: PVCs fall simultaneously with the upstroke or peak of the T wave of the previous beat.

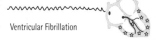

Sustained Ventricular Tachycardia
Tachycardia with broad QRS complexes at a rate of > 90 beats/min.

Ventricular Tachycardia

DD: supraventricular tachycardia with BBB.

Ventricular Fibrillation
Chaotic ventricular electrical discharge.

Ventricular Fibrillation

Long QT Syndrome
Abnormal prolongation of the corrected QT Interval.

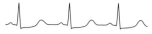

Carditis, Cardiomyopathy

Acute Pericarditis
Simultaneous ST elevations over the anterior and posterior wall, typically originating from the S wave. Can be misinterpreted as a myocardial infarction.

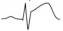

Hypertrophic (Obstructive) Cardiomyopathy
Signs of left ventricular hypertrophy (Sokolow index), varying ST segment changes (depressions, elevations) without classic localization, deep inverted T waves.

Dilated Cardiomyopathy
Nonspecific repolarization disturbances, bundle branch like pictures and arrhythmias.

Electrolyte Disturbances, Drugs

Hypokalemia
Repolarization disorders, ST depressions, prominent U waves, may merge into TU wave.

Hyperkalemia
Tall, peaked T waves that later flatten, broad QRS complex. Finally tachycardic arrhythmias can occur resulting in bradycardia and asystole.

Hypercalcemia
Shortening of the corrected QT Interval (QTc).

Hypocalcemia
Prolongation of the QT Interval.

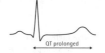

ECG Changes induced by Digitalis
Shallow ST depressions, AV blocks possible.

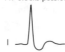

ECG Evaluation Sheet

Patient
Initials ___ Date of birth ␣␣|␣␣day|␣ 1 9 ␣␣|␣year Sex ☐ F ☐ M
Main diagnosis: _____
Antiarrhythmics: _____ Digitalis ○

RR Intervals Regular Y N

Heart Rate ____ / min Tachycardia (> 90/min) ○ Bradycardia (< 50/min) ○

P Wave
Positive in I, II, III (sinus rhythm) Y N
Regular, followed by QRS Y N — absolute arrhythmia (atrial fibrillation) ○
"sawtooth" (atrial flutter) ○

PR Interval 0.12 – 0.20 s Y N — shortened, < 0.12 s ○ prolonged, > 0.2 s (AV block) ○

Axis Deviation
$S_I Q_{III}$ pattern ○ ($S_I S_{II} S_{III}$ pattern) ○ Extreme axis deviation ○
Left axis deviation ○ Right axis deviation ○
Normal ○

QRS Complex QRS duration normal < 0.1 s Y N — Incomplete bundle branch block (0.10 – 0.12 s) ○
Complete bundle branch block (> 0.12 s) ○
Terminal deflection delayed in V_1 (> 0.03 s)→ RBBB ○
Terminal deflection delayed in V_6 (> 0.05 s)→ LBBB ○

R Progression Normal in $V_1 – V_6$ Y N — insufficient R Progression in ○ ○ ○ ○ ○ ○
V_1 V_2 V_3 V_4 V_5 V_6

Q Wave Significantly pathological in N Y — ○ ○ ○ ○ ○ ○ ○ ○ ○
V_1 V_2 V_3 V_4 V_5 V_6 II III aVF

Signs of Hypertrophy N Y — $S_{V2} + R_{V5} > 3.5$ mV (Sokolov le.) ○ $R_{V2} + S_{V5} > 1.05$ mV (Sokolov ri.) ○

ST Segment Isoelectric Y N — ST elevation in ○ ○ ○ ○ ○ ○ ○ ○ ○ ○ ○
V_1 V_2 V_3 V_4 V_5 V_6 I II III aVR aVL aVF
ST depression in ○ ○ ○ ○ ○ ○ ○ ○ ○ ○ ○ ○
V_1 V_2 V_3 V_4 V_5 V_6 I II III aVR aVL aVF
ascend. ○ horizont. ○ descend. ○

T Wave Positive in I – III, V_1–V_4 Y N — negative T wave symmetr. ○ preterminal ○ terminal ○

QT Interval QT_C normal Y N QT interval: __.__ Corrected QT interval (QT_C) __.__ Bazett: $\dfrac{QT (s)}{\sqrt{RR (s)}}$
(0.40–0.44)

Evaluation (ECG Diagnosis)
_____

Normal ○ Borderline ○ Pathological ○

© 1997-2002
Börm Bruckmeier Publishing LLC
www.media4u.com

Signature _____ Date ␣␣|␣month|␣day| 2 0 ␣␣

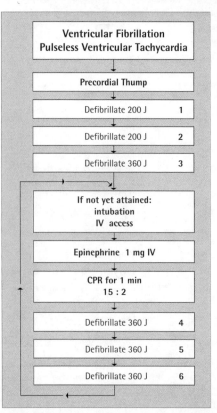

Ventricular Fibrillation
Pulseless Ventricular Tachycardia

↓

Precordial Thump

↓

Defibrillate 200 J   1

↓

Defibrillate 200 J   2

↓

Defibrillate 360 J   3

↓

If not yet attained:
intubation
IV access

↓

Epinephrine 1 mg IV

↓

CPR for 1 min
15 : 2

↓

Defibrillate 360 J   4

↓

Defibrillate 360 J   5

↓

Defibrillate 360 J   6

Emergency Guidelines in Ventricular Tachycardia and Ventricular Fibrillation

Myocardial Infarction: Localization, Stages

Infarct Localization											
	I	II	III	aVL	aVF	rV4	V2	V3	V4	V5	V6
apical	+			+			+	+	+		
anteroseptal							+	+			.
anterolateral	+			+						+	+
posterolateral			+		+					+	+
inferior		+	+		+						
right ventricular			+		+	+	(+)				

Stage	Age	ECG	Criteria
early stage	> a few minutes		high T waves
stage I	up to 6 hours		ST elevation R preserved no/small Q wave
intermed. stage	> 6 hours		ST elevation with T wave inversion loss of R wave, infarct Q
stage II	days		infarct Q T wave inversion ST normalization
stage III	residual		persistant Q loss of R wave T normalization

Normogram of QT Interval, Bazett Formula

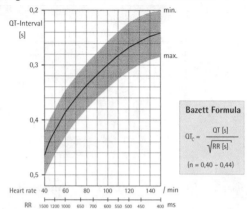

Bazett Formula

$$QT_c = \frac{QT\ [s]}{\sqrt{RR\ [s]}}$$

(n = 0,40 – 0,44)

Normal Intervals, Sokolow Index

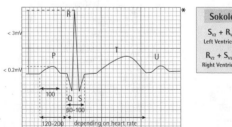

Sokolow Index

$S_{V2} + R_{V5} > 3{,}5\ mV$
Left Ventricular Hypertrophy

$R_{V2} + S_{V5} > 1{,}05\ mV$
Right Ventricular Hypertrophy

Cardiac Axis, Lewis Cycle

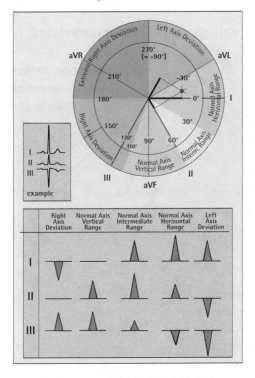

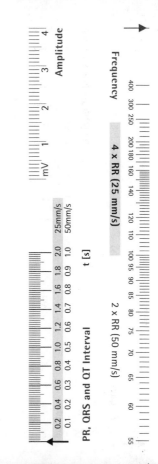

Frequency

400 300 250 200 180 160 140 120 110 100 95 90 85 80 75 70 65 60 55

4 x RR (25 mm/s)

2 x RR (50 mm/s)

Amplitude

4

3

2

1

mV

t [s]

25mm/s
50mm/s

2.0 1.8 1.6 1.4 1.2 1.0 0.8 0.6 0.4 0.2
1.0 0.9 0.8 0.7 0.6 0.5 0.4 0.3 0.2 0.1

PR, QRS and QT Interval

ECG Ruler
Cut it out!

Better: ECG Ruler pocketcard
→ www.media4u.com

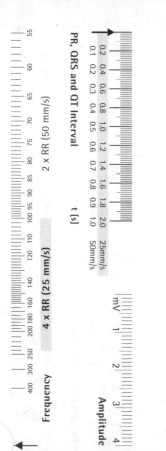

PR, QRS and QT Interval

2 x RR (50 mm/s)

t [s]

0.1 0.2 0.3 0.4 0.5 0.6 0.7 0.8 0.9 1.0
0.2 0.4 0.6 0.8 1.0 1.2 1.4 1.6 1.8 2.0

25mm/s
50mm/s

55 60 65 70 75 80 85 90 95 100 110 120 140 160 180 200 250 300 400

4 x RR (25 mm/s)

Frequency

mV 1 2 3 4

Amplitude

ECG Ruler
Cut it out!

Better: ECG Ruler pocketcard
→ www.media4u.com

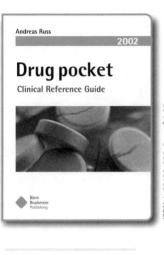
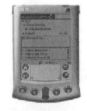

◆ Börm Bruckmeier Publishing

Internet: www.media4u.com	**Fax:** 419-281-6883 **Phone:** 888-322-6657	**Mail:** Börm Bruckmeier Publishing PO Box 388 Ashland, OH 44805

Name

Address

E-mail

City   State   Zip

	COPIES		PRICE/COPY		PRICE
Drug pocket 2002		x	$ 9.95	=	
Differential Diagnosis pocket		x	$12.95	=	
ECG pocket		x	$12.95	=	
Medical Spanish pocket		x	$12.95	=	
Antibiotics pocketcard 2002		x	$ 3.95	=	
BLS/ALS pocketcard		x	$ 3.95	=	
ECG pocketcard		x	$ 3.95	=.	
ECG Evaluation pocketcard		x	$ 3.95	=	
ECG Ruler pocketcard		x	$ 3.95	=	
ECG pocketcards (set of 3 cards)		x	$ 9.95	=	
Emergency Drugs pocketcard		x	$ 3.95	=	
H&P pocketcard		x	$ 3.95	=	
Medical Abbreviations pocketcard (2 cards)		x	$ 6.95	=	
Medical Spanish pocketcard		x	$ 3.95	=	
Neurology pocketcard (2 cards)		x	$ 6.95	=	
Normal Values pocketcard		x	$ 3.95	=	

Sales Tax: CA residents add 8%, OH 6.25%

Shipping & Handling for US addresses:
UPS Standard: 10% of subtotal (minimum $5.00)
UPS 2nd Day Air: 20% of subtotal (minimum $8.00)

Credit Card: ☐ Visa ☐ Mastercard ☐ Amex ☐ Discover
Card Number

Exp. Date   Signature

= **Subtotal**
+ Sales Tax
+ S&H

= **Total**

For foreign orders, volume discount, shipping and payment questions, please contact us at: service@media4u.com